How to Operate Your Body

THE LEGS

Fiction books by William C. Tracy

The Dissolutionverse:
Novellas and Novelettes:
The Five Hive Plateau
Tuning the Symphony
Merchants and Maji
The Society of Two Houses
Journey to the Top of the Nether

The Dissolution Cycle:
The Seeds of Dissolution (Book I)
Facets of the Nether (Book II)
Fall of the Imperium (Book III)

Epic Fantasy:
Fruits of the Gods

Anthologies:
Distant Gardens
Farther Reefs
The World of Juno

Science Fiction
The Biomass Conflux
Of Mycelium and Men
Down Among the Mushrooms
To a Fungus Unknown
The Spores of Wrath

How to Operate Your Body

THE LEGS

William C. Tracy

Space Wizard Science Fantasy
Raleigh, NC
www.spacewizardsciencefantasy.com

Cover Design by MoorBooks
Editing by Heather Tracy
Book Layout © 2015 BookDesignTemplates.com
Pictures copyright Josiah Brooks and William C. Tracy
All Gray's Anatomy illustrations are open source.

How to Operate Your Body/William C. Tracy.— 1st ed.
ISBN 978-1-960247-17-9

Author's website: spacewizardsciencefantasy.com

Dedicated to all those Sunday practice sessions.

CONTENTS

Foreword

This is your meat-bag.
No one gave you a manual.
Let's learn how it works.

There is a simple revelation in the haiku above: life does not, in fact, give you a manual. However, we as humans have conquered many challenges. We've created and recorded vast stores of knowledge. We have redefined ourselves and continue to advance in math, science, engineering, history, art, law, etc.

We will spend months or years learning a new skill. We pride ourselves on learning some piece of newly invented technology. But very few of us spend time learning how our bodies operate. But are our bodies not our own, personal, machines? We will learn how to modify our computers and upgrade them. We buy the latest new technology or games to get that new thrill, but when a part of our body underperforms, we just run to a doctor or shrug it off.

Your body is as capable as the newest technology. It's time to make it better, faster, stronger.

I'm William C. Tracy, and I've spent the last twenty years working in the field of body mechanics. I have a master's in mechanical engineering, specializing in linkage dynamics, and have been active in martial arts since 2002. The two fields may not seem related, but together they allowed for a journey of investigation into how my body operates mechanically, energetically, and practically.

Now, some twenty years later, I have many years as a performance engineer at a major construction company behind me. During that time, I worked on kinematic systems (how things move with and against each other), and control systems (keeping complex systems in balance). I've worked nearly as long teaching martial arts.

In the past decade, I received instruction from some really excellent martial artists, including: Hironori Otsuka III, the grandmaster of Wado Ryu Karate (my style); David Gimberline, an instructor of Shotokan, Shoto Ryu, Goshin Justsu, and practical karate applications; and Elmar Schmeisser, a karate instructor with over fifty years of experience in multiple martial arts disciplines, as well as neurophysiology.

After learning with these instructors, I focused on the fine methods of control for each musculature system in the body, incorporating them into my teaching style.

But in this book, I'm not going to teach you martial arts, how to punch, kick, or how to attack people. Instead, I'm going to teach you how to *move*.

Moving—putting one foot in front of the other, reaching, stretching, or just getting out of the bed in the morning—is not something we often think about. But it's incredibly important. Many causes of bad backs, sore legs and tight necks lie in poor posture and inefficient movement.

However, that's not the biggest thing this book will teach you. It will teach you how to move *efficiently*. There is a big difference in efficient motion and just moving.

Periodically, I'll ask you to do exercises. If you follow along and try them out, you'll have a much better time understanding what I'm saying. My advice is to do them, even if you think you understand the principles already. One of my favorite moments in martial arts is when a student starts practicing a simple concept I've nagged them about for years, then is surprised it works! Really, try things out and I think you'll be surprised.

To temper that, I have a quick *I Am Not a Doctor* warning. Much of the knowledge presented in this book comes from experimentation and observation over many years, but I don't have a degree or license in physical therapy, or medicine. I'll give you, the reader, the warning I give my karate students: **don't do something if it hurts**. Human bodies are all different, with large ranges of shapes and flexibilities. If an exercise I suggest hurts or seems impossible for you, don't do it! Use your own discretion, especially if you have a specific limitation.

Finally, if these explanations and examples help you, please pass them on to others! There's no secret to this. It's simply a lot of observation and trial and error. I hope to ease a little pain, smooth a little frustration, and help people live to their full potential. Bad backs, achy knees, stiff necks, no longer! Let's learn How to Operate Your Body.

William C. Tracy
April 2023

Correct posture

Hips, Shoulders, Back, Knees, Feet, and Head

Operating your body well is no easy matter. Imagine that you are an infant. You don't know how to move your arms or your legs, or really how to do anything. Pretend you are discovering your body's limits for the very first time. It's much easier to learn something new rather than relearn, but coming at a new technique with an open mind helps bridge that gap.

One of the core problems, and one of the most easily corrected issues with body mechanics, is posture. Having good posture is essential to learning concepts introduced later in this book, like how to walk efficiently. Seriously, if you keep only one lesson from this book, work on posture.

We often get so used to doing an action a certain way that it feels alien to do it any other way. I may ask you to undo something you're used to, or at least try a different method. It's as uncomfortable as eating or brushing your teeth with your non-

So, you want to feel better and get in shape, right? Does your back hurt when you play video games, or do your hips ache after a day at the office? This is the book for you! Instead of telling you what weights to lift at the gym, this book will give you some simple exercises to get you feeling better and moving quicker. After you're moving efficiently, then you can decide if you want to hit the gym!

dominant hand. But give it a try. At least by changing your posture you won't get toothpaste all over your face.

Before we get to how to operate your legs correctly, we're going to build up some good habits to make the final section of this book easier to understand. Stay with me and I promise we'll get there!

With each new section you go through in this book, you will feel differences in posture, body connections from your feet to your shoulders, and of course, how you walk. Take the time to really understand what's going on, and when each change starts to gel, then it's time to move on to the next section.

For learning posture, let's take this from the head down. The bulbous cabbage sitting on top of your shoulders can weigh as much as a bowling ball. If this bowling ball is sticking out in front of you, rather than being directly above your body, you'll be predisposed to moving where the bowling ball leads you.

First exercise! If you have a bowling ball, use that, but if not, get something else that weighs about 15 pounds (that's about 7 kg for those using the metric system). Hold the object directly in front of you, cradling it with your hands, touching your stomach around your bellybutton. You'll feel the weight, but it probably won't be too much of an imposition. That's because where you're holding it is very close to your center of mass.

Ah. I should step back and explain the center of mass.

If you want to be technical about it, the way to find the center of mass is this: take an object, wrap it with a piece of string from one end to another, then hang it up on a wall. Draw a line along the length of the string. Now, take the same object, wrap the string around a different length, and hang it up again a different way. Draw another line. If you do this several different times, the center of mass will be where all the lines cross. Let's use Vitty the Vitruvian Man as an example. You can see in Figure 1 how the vertical line describes his center of mass when hung up in different directions.

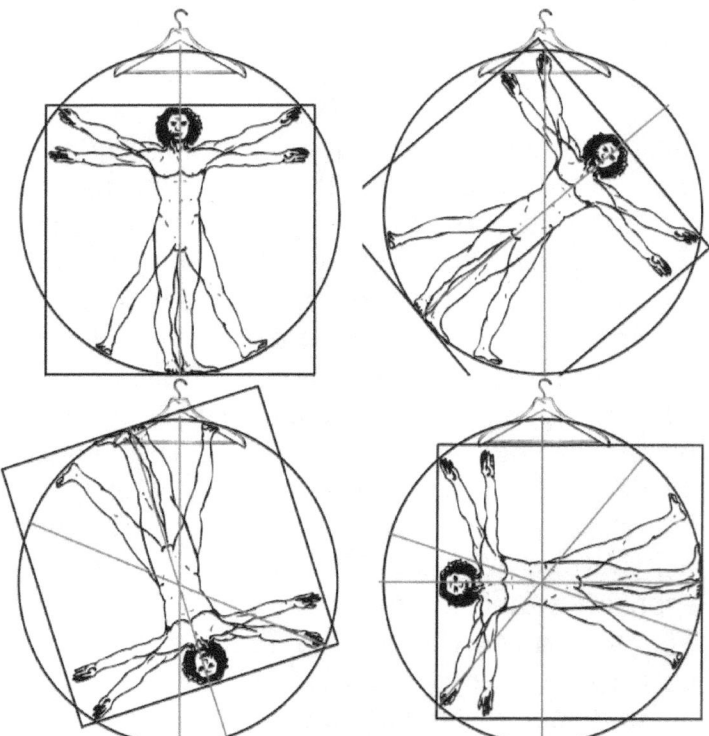

Figure 1: Vitty is hung up by his head, arms, legs, and side to determine his center of mass.

Granted, you're probably not going to wrap yourself up in string and tape yourself to the wall. If you do, please send me pictures.

For now, take my word for it that your center of mass—assuming you own two arms, two legs, your head, and you're standing upright—is right around your bellybutton.

So, you're standing there with a bowling ball held at your center of mass. You're still holding the bowling ball, right? No? Well, pick it up again.

As I said, when you hold this at your center of mass, it doesn't affect your balance much because the mass is concentrated where you carry mass all the time. Try reaching your hands out so your elbows are at your stomach and the bowling ball is out in front of you. It feels a lot heavier, doesn't it? Now, try lifting the ball up so you're holding it at the same height as your head, directly in front of you. You feel like you're going to fall forward, right? Now you can put the ball down.

When you stand upright and your head is not directly above your body, the situation is the same as holding a bowling ball in front of your face. You're predisposed to moving forward, rather than any other direction. But since you're used to doing so, you don't notice your body's bias. To be able to move efficiently, you want to start from a true neutral stance. Let's continue correcting that bias.

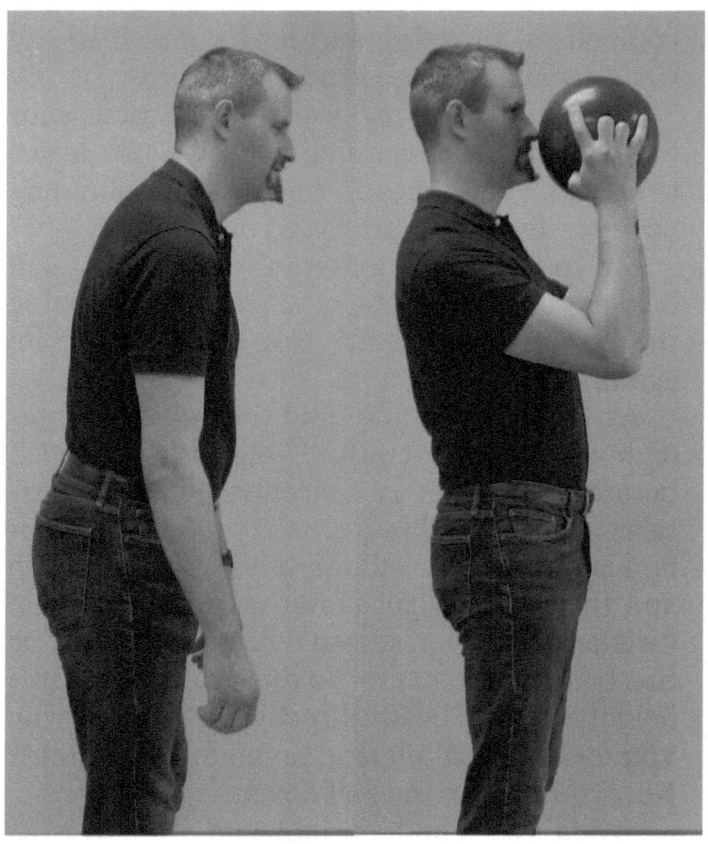

Figure 2: A bowling ball held in front of your head simulates the weight of keeping your head forward.

Second exercise. Bring your head back so your ears are directly above your shoulders. Make sure you don't raise your chin when you do this (and don't push your shoulders forward either!). Keep your eyes level so you're not looking down your nose. You may feel a slight pressure in your neck if it's not used to this position. If you're standing up, you may even start to tip backward because you're used to holding your head forward all the time. Not falling over means you're learning to compensate for standing up straight.

If I had to guess, I'd suspect after moving your head into a strange position, your shoulders are now bunched up near your ears. Next step, relax your shoulders.

Keep your ears above your shoulders, or rather above the center of your body. While you do this, bring your shoulders up to your ears, like I just said not to. Then push them all the way back as far as they can go. Last, bring your shoulders straight down. To recap, up into your ears, straight back, straight down. This is where your shoulders should be. It may feel like you're really pushing them backward, but again, that's because you're used to keeping them forward.

If your shoulders are tight, they may crackle when you move them up, back, and down. That's just the synovial fluid getting released from where it's been pent up. Don't worry about it.

Where's your head?

Has it gone forward again? Are you holding a bowling ball up in the air?

Now we have two pieces to put together. Fix your shoulders as above, then fix your head so your ears are above your shoulders. Your chest will protrude when you do this, no matter your gender. That's because this is correct posture. You already look more confident and authoritative. I've used both correct posture and incorrect posture in groups of people. They take more notice and defer to you when you have correct head and shoulder posture. It's as if we know as a social group that if someone can get this detail right, they may know what they're talking about.

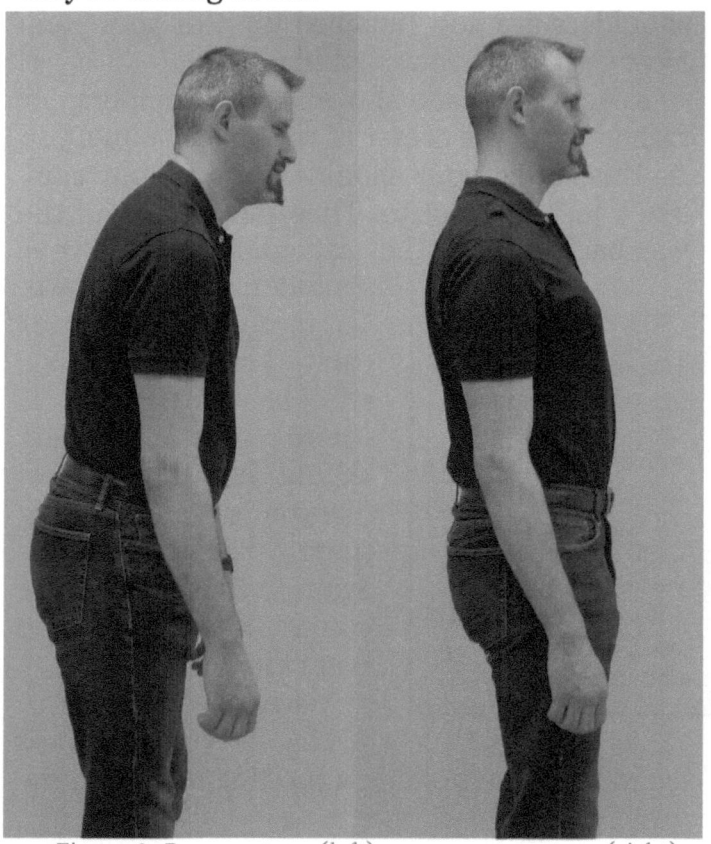

Figure 3: Poor posture (left) vs. correct posture (right). We pay more attention to people with good posture.

Okay, we've fixed the top half, but what about the rest? Positioning your upper body directly over your legs will make it much easier to walk more efficiently.

If your lower back hurts, you might be compressing it with poor posture. This part is going to be a little hard to explain, but I'll do my best.

How often do you pay attention to your hips? The answer is: not enough (yes, I'm aware I'm making an assumption...I'm also aware I'm correct). Remember when I talked about your center of mass? What joint is closest to that area? Your hips. Fixing the way your hips work can improve your posture, fix back problems, improve your gait, and much more.

The biggest problem I see with my introductory martial arts students is that their hips are all wrong. The way most of us naturally stand is with our butts pushed out behind us. This is a "lazy" posture. It's lazy because you're not using your muscles. When you stand this way, you can "lock" your lower back, then you don't have to use your core muscles or your back muscles to help you stand. Sure, it takes less energy muscle-wise, but it also puts more strain on the bones and disks of your spine. It's not a coincidence back problems are one of the most common of the human body. If you're not used to keeping a connection in your core, don't worry. I'll get to that in a few chapters.

Try the "lazy" position out, if you don't naturally stand that way. Stand straight, push your butt out, and let your belly relax. Now stop doing it. Since you've experienced this posture, you can do the opposite.

Instead of pushing your butt out behind you, tuck your hips inward. If you have trouble feeling this, try the following: Put your hands on your hips. Align the edge of your forefinger with the vertical seam of your pants. The more you stick your butt out, the more your finger is going to point behind you. What you want to do is bring your finger so it points straight down.

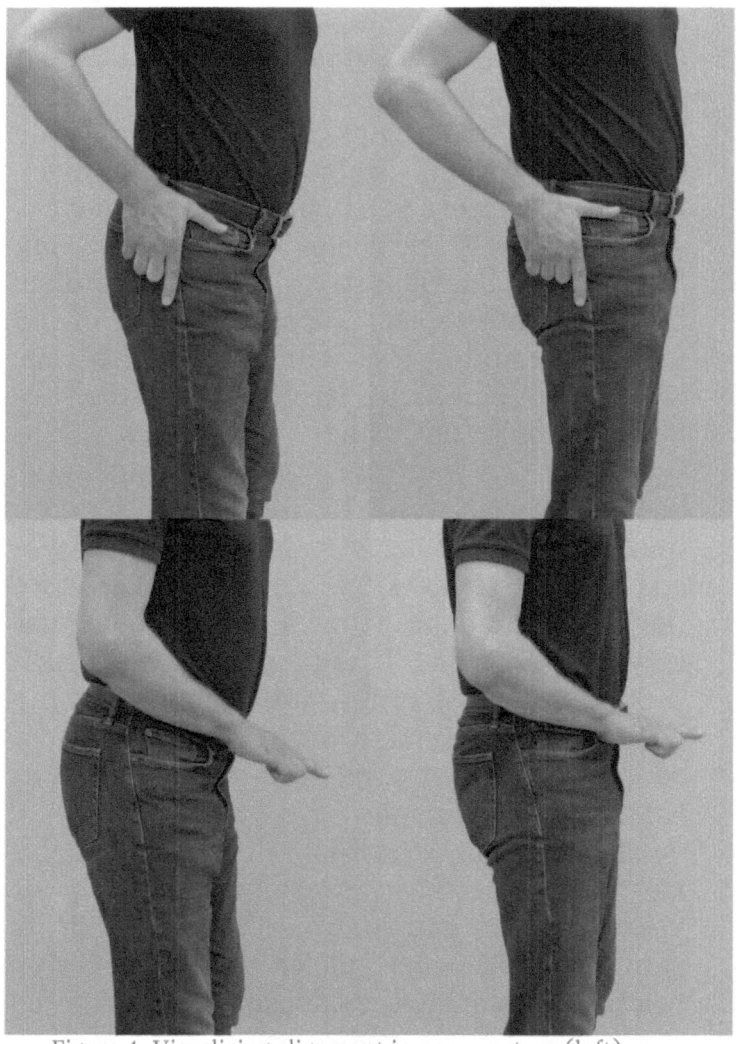

Figure 4: Visualizing alignment in poor posture (left) vs. correct posture (right).

If that doesn't work for you, here's another way to visualize it. Point your forefinger straight out from the button that fastens your pants. Or if you're wearing a belt, straight out from the buckle. Not straight out parallel to the floor, but straight in the direction the button or belt buckle is pointing.

If you're sticking your butt out, then your finger will be pointing slightly down. You want to tuck your hips in until your finger is pointing parallel to the ground. As you do this, you may feel your back lengthen. This is a good sign.

Let's put the three exercises together. Are you holding a bowling ball (or object of similar weight) too far forward? First bring your head back so your ears are above your center of mass. Tuck your chin. Second, get those shoulders out of your ears. Up, back, and down. Third, tuck your hips in so your belt buckle is pointing straight forward. You're well on the way to good posture.

Along with your hips, it's also important to pay attention to your knees. You shouldn't ever lock them out. First, this can hyperextend your knee (that is, extend it more than it should, which will stress your joints), and second, straight knees keep you from adjusting your balance on the fly. Adjusting balance is something we all do naturally. This is partially what makes the Boston dynamics robots' movement seem so natural (or scary). We see a robot kicked, stumble, and right its balance, just as we can. They've managed to program a robot to bend its knees. This will be our downfall.

But you too can bend your knees and fight the robot menace! Flexing your knees just a little engages your thigh muscles and lets you react faster to anything that would push you off balance. If you add this to the other three tips above, you will not only have better posture, but be able to hold it better and for longer.

If you do have lower back problems, there's another exercise to help you lengthen your back and stretch it out.

With your good balance (head, shoulders, hips, knees), turn your feet slightly inward (no more than about ten degrees), and let your knees and your hips follow them. Keep your knees above your toes. This opens up your lower back area. While tucking your hips as well as turning your legs toward each other, your back will stretch in two directions. You can add a third stretch if you think about extending outward rather than compressing inward. Pretend your head is tied to the ceiling by a piece of string, keep your body taut. Reach upward with your head (in good posture, yes).

Now, it's time to practice. Set a timer for thirty seconds or set a "good posture reminder" on your phone, if needed. I'm not joking when I suggest every thirty seconds. Or even less. It's at once satisfying and frustrating to feel how much you can straighten up. When your shoulders and neck and hips open up,

Up to now, I've shown you what to do, but here's the really hard part. Unless you actually practice correct posture, you won't do it.

everything will feel much better. But you'll naturally sag back to a "lazy" posture after a few moments.

You'll feel it every single time your timer goes off, but over time your posture will improve.

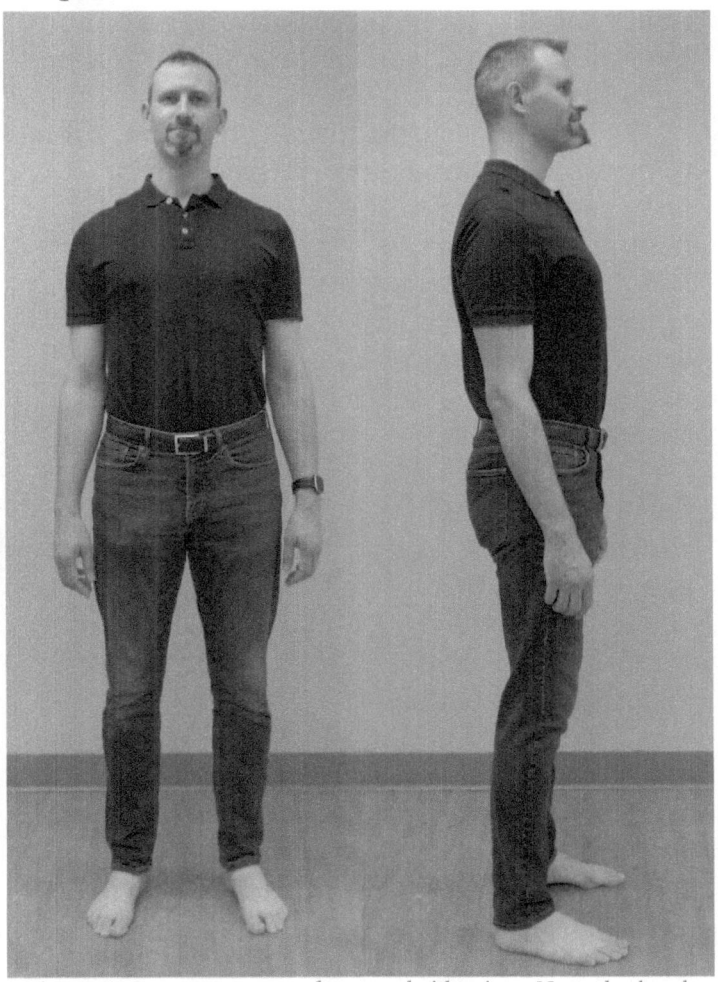

Figure 5: Correct posture, front and side view. Note the head is extended upward, as if connected to the ceiling with string.

I promise it will get easier. The more often you remind yourself to have good posture, and follow through with the exercise above, the more often your body will naturally line up in that position. Over time, you'll be able to increase the reminder time to a minute, two minutes, five ten, half an hour, and more. Eventually, you'll wonder how you ever stood up before.

We'll leave basic posture for now, but I'll be referencing it throughout this book. For now, just keep these four points in mind: *head, shoulders, hips, knees*. You can adjust these while standing or sitting. Try both! If I reference one of these four or tell you to get back to good posture, you'll understand what I mean. You just thought about it again, didn't you? Go ahead and fix your posture one more time before the next section!

At this point, you're likely wondering, "isn't this book supposed to be about legs?" Yes. Yes, it is. But it will take time to get there. You're balancing the rest of your body *on* your legs. We're making sure the above-the-legs part doesn't interfere while you learn to walk.

Learning about your center

I talked briefly about your center above, but I want to go more in depth. Whether you call this your center, your bellybutton, your center of mass, the center of your chi, your tanden or hara, your Dantian, your sacral or svadhishthna chakra, etcetera—people have recognized the significance of this area for thousands of years. It makes sense that it has some importance tied to it. I'm going to leave aside all the metaphysical implications as that could fill another book and I'm not the correct person to write it.

Instead, I'm going to talk about the physical and mechanical aspects of your center. I say your bellybutton, or refer to your hips moving, but the actual position is about three fingers down from your bellybutton and two fingers inside your body. This is that spot you would find if you hung yourself up a wall with string like Vitty in the last section.

Now you know how to find your center of mass, but why would you want to? Have you ever balanced a pen or spoon or fork on one finger before? You can do this because you are finding its center of mass. The unique property of the center of mass of an object is that if you manipulate the center, you will manipulate the entire object at one time. This is assuming the object you are manipulating is rigid, or at least does not flex too much. Obviously, your body flexes a lot, as you can move your arms and legs and head in all directions. For right now I'm talking about your center when your feet are both planted on the floor, about as wide apart as your hips, you have good posture as outlined above (remember your posture!), and your hands are hanging by your sides.

How do you get to know your center? First you need to have good posture. I know I keep harping on this, but it really is important. Changing your posture will change where your center of mass is. You want your physical center of mass to line up with your meta-physical one (three fingers down and two fingers in from your bellybutton). Feet at hip width, knees slightly bent, hips tucked, shoulders back and down, ears in line with your shoulders. Extend your body as if your head is hanging by a string from the ceiling.

If you get really good at finding the center of objects, you can do astounding feats like balancing circular objects on top of one another, or juggling six or seven balls, or doing several complicated actions at once. That takes a lot of practice, although it is fun to do.

Whew! That's a lot. But keep at it. Getting into that position will become second nature, especially if you keep doing it every time I mention it while you read this book. Do you have a timer running?

In good posture, your center is aligned. Now let's play with it. We are going to move different body parts around to show you how much effect it has on your center. First, from good position, put both arms out in front of you, relaxed, at the height of your shoulders, as if you've become a zombie and want a brain sandwich. Then push both shoulders forward and reach out as far as you can with your hands. Get those brains! As you do this you'll start toppling forward. Reset and try it again. Feel free to stagger and moan and see if anyone hits you with a baseball bat.

The arms are the easiest to try this exercise with, because they make the largest change in your center of mass from a standing position. Let's try two others and see if you can feel the difference. Get back in a good posture (remember to tuck those hips!), and start leaning your head forward, as if you are a turtle poking out of your shell. This simulates holding that bowling ball in front of your face. You may have to go farther than you would using your arms before you start falling forward, because your head doesn't reach as far (I hope!).

One more. Get back in a good position, especially making sure to tuck your hips under you, because this is what we're going to move. Start pointing your pants button or belt buckle downward and stick your butt out, and feel when you begin falling backward. If you've got a "lazy" posture, this is the difference you have to contend with while walking around. It's quite significant.

The reason these small motions make such a difference is because you are aligned with your center of mass and, like balancing a pencil on your finger, you have very fine control over your body. These are simple examples, and you can play on your own by adjusting both your posture, and where your arms and legs are.

I'll get to more applications of controlled movement later in the book, but for now pay attention to a few things while you move around, at least until you're comfortable with good posture. The first is that when you are aligned over your center, in good posture, you will be lighter on your feet. This happens because you don't have to account for being off balance while your head is forward or your hips are misaligned. Second, try things like walking up hills while you have good posture. I bet it will be easier! I'll leave you to play with this for now, but I'll come back to it again at the end of the book. For now, don't lose your posture! Head, shoulders, hips, knees.

> You'll find your balance gets a lot better when your center is aligned. For example, standing on one foot is a lot easier with good posture.

In fact, if you've read up to here from the beginning, this is a good place to take a break before we get to more complicated actions. Practice standing with your timer. See if you can get up to 30 seconds without losing your posture. Do you have good posture both while standing and sitting? Are your shoulders relaxed? Remember what I said at the beginning of this chapter: If you only take one thing away from this book, take this one. Good posture will fix a lot of things by itself.

Moving Around

Muscles, Ligaments and Tendons

Now you understand a bit about how your body is affected by your posture and center of mass, I want to talk about the way your body is internally connected. You've probably heard this in high school biology, so I'm not going to go too in-depth.

In this section, we're going to cover anatomy from your feet to your abdomen. All these body parts are used together when walking. This is why these explanations are in a book about your legs!

First, muscles. Basically, muscles are a soft tissue made of protein, where strands slide past each other so the muscle can contract and release. These are the things that connect your bones together and enable you to stand up. Without them, you wouldn't be able to move and would collapse in a pile.

There are several different types of muscle, including cardiac muscle in your heart, the smooth muscle in your internal organs, and skeletal muscle—that is the muscle that binds your skeleton together. The first two muscle types are largely involuntary. That is, you have no control over them. Instead, let's talk about where you *do* have control. Having control means you can improve in those areas, especially if you haven't tried before.

Learning how your muscles move is the basis for understanding how to operate your body. Play around with how your body moves. Open and close your hands. See how it affects your forearm. Move your foot up and down, and see how it affects your lower leg and calf. Sit and stand while you put your hands on your butt, to see how your gluteus muscles contract and expand. Basically, go touch yourself a lot (not a euphemism). You'll learn some things.

Two other types of tissue that are intertwined (literally) with muscles are ligaments and tendons. People often confuse these, if they even know what they are. If you've ever seen an anatomy diagram, you usually see a muscle colored in red. You also may see another bit of something colored in white that attaches to or emerges from the muscle. This is usually the connective tendon.

Tendons are tough bands of tissue, sort of like rubber bands, and while they don't contract and expand as much as muscle fibers do, they are the things that let your muscles work with your skeleton. A tendon emerges from a muscle and connects to one of the nearby bones, acting as an anchor. Imagine you have a bunch of bones, and you want to figure out how to make them move around. You could blow up a balloon halfway so that the shape is malleable—long and thin or short and round. This is sort of how a muscle moves. But then how do you connect that balloon to your bones? Cut a rubber band, tie one end around the neck of the balloon, and tie the other end around one of the bones. Tape the top of the balloon to another bone. The rubber band lets the balloon flex. You have the equivalent of a tendon. Tendons are tough, can resist a lot of stress, but can tear if they are moved in the wrong direction or stretched too far. The Achilles tendon is one of the easiest ones to find in your body. Sit down and bring one foot up in front of you, or rest it on your other leg. Put your thumb on the area between your heel and your ankle, then move your foot up and down. You'll feel a thick band there that tenses and relaxes as you move your foot. If you move your fingers up your leg, you can feel how the Achilles tendon interacts with your muscle all the way up to your calf, right below your knee. So, tendons are like thick rubber bands

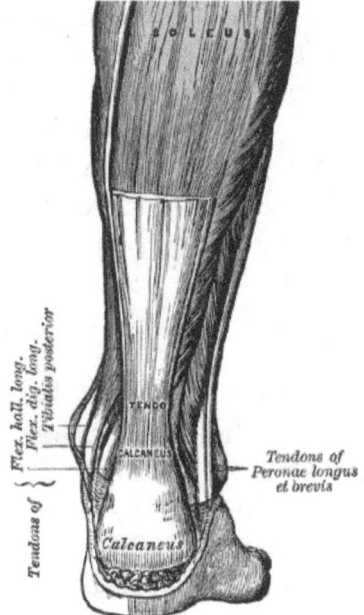

Figure 6: The Achilles Tendon (*Gray's Anatomy*).

attaching muscle to bone.

Ligaments, on the other hand (or *in* the other hand, right? Right?), are much more static than tendons, because ligaments connect bones to other bones. There is little expansion and contraction like there is in a muscle. Just like a tendon, a ligament can be torn from an injury, from overexertion, or for moving your body in a way that it's not supposed to move. If you want to feel a ligament, again sit down, but this time put both feet on the floor. Put a hand on one knee and let your fingers rest right beneath your kneecap. You will feel a thick band of tissue. If you swing your lower leg up then back to the floor, you can feel this band of tissue as it flexes a small amount between your leg bone and your kneecap. It doesn't move nearly as much as your Achilles tendon does. Ligaments don't move as much as tendons because bones generally stay in the same place in our bodies, unlike muscles. However, ligaments also take longer to heal because your bones grow a lot slower than your muscles do. What you're feeling under your kneecap is the patellar ligament (often called the patellar tendon, but that's technically wrong, and now you know why!)

Behind that, *inside* your knee is yet another ligament. If you've heard of someone with a torn ACL, that's the anterior cruciate *ligament*, and it will often never repair on its own, instead needing surgery. Don't mess around with your ligaments. You need them!

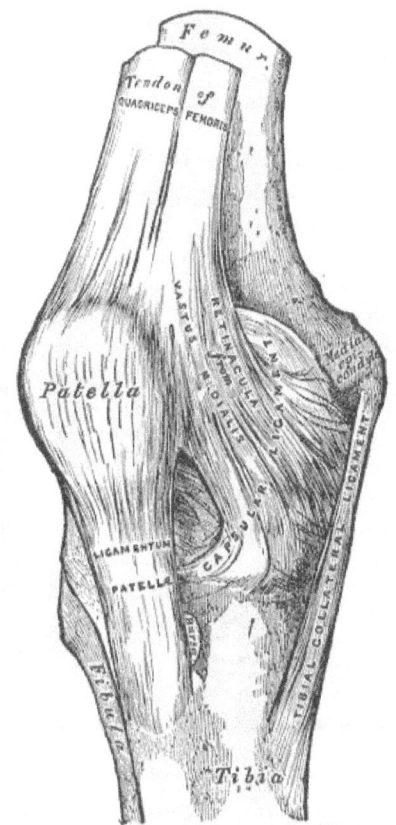

Figure 7: The patellar ligament (*Gray's Anatomy*). The ACL is inside the knee joint, connecting the femur and tibia.

Again, I encourage you to feel your own body. Where a part of you bends (arms, legs, waist, neck, etc.), put a hand on the area that moves the most as you bend. You can feel all these little connections. A great example is your shoulder, because it moves in all directions. Put a hand on your opposite shoulder and move your arm around. You'll feel a bunch of muscles, tendons, and ligaments all moving in your shoulder joint.

Discovering what's happening is one of the best ways to learn how to operate your body.

Changing the way your body moves, especially if you're adopting a new way of standing (with correct posture), can lead to more stress on muscles that aren't used to the load. You might find your shoulders or back hurt *more* the first few days of using correct posture. As always, make certain what you are doing is correct posture, and you're not introducing a new imbalance or compensation. It's ok to take breaks from this new posture but try to add a little more time each day. Soon you'll get used to it, and I promise good posture will lead to fewer aches and pains in the long run. A good way to make that happen sooner is in the next section.

The importance of small muscles

The little muscles or support muscles are vitally important to having a well-balanced body. Many fitness books, weightlifting programs, and even some personal trainers skip over this, but it's dangerous to do so. These small sections of larger muscles help out as you move, providing stabilization and control. If you are trying to increase your muscle mass (which is by no means required to get a lot out of this book), a lot of training programs will focus on making the big muscles bigger, because they're more impressive aesthetically. However, big muscles without a good support staff can lead to joint problems in the future. It's like trying to run a large business with only a CEO. You need employees to support and carry out the decisions made by the person at the top.

Instead of being able to lift a large weight in one direction, I've found it's more useful to lift a normal or light weight in *any* direction with full control. Jugglers don't juggle extremely heavy objects, except for quick stunts with bowling balls and chainsaws. Usually, they use light balls or pins. They develop full control over them. If you watch an accomplished juggler walk around or do tricks while still juggling several balls, and wonder how they do that, *this* is how. They have small muscular control. Be like the juggler. Once you have developed small muscles, then work on making the big muscles bigger if you wish. With large muscles buoyed by a support staff of small muscles, you have a much-reduced chance of joint injury. As I've detailed above, you *really* don't want to have an injured joint. Tendons take a long time to heal. Ligaments may never heal without surgery. They are one of the worst injuries to have, especially in an active sport. While bones heal and can

> Unless you are already used to lifting heavy weights—which most people aren't—you might find a different type of exercise more helpful. Performing slow, controlled exercises can be very beneficial.

even become denser with trauma, ligaments and tendons take an agonizingly long time to heal—on the order of months or even years.

Here are a couple simple exercises to show you—even if you are used to lifting a lot of weight—how useful it is to develop small muscle mass.

Wall push-ups: stand a couple feet out from a wall, facing it. Raise your arms so you can comfortably place your palms on the wall, while allowing just a little bit of flex in your elbows. Remember your good posture from the first chapter! Get your shoulders back, your head back, and tuck your hips in. Now, while keeping all those parts in alignment, slowly bend your elbows to bring your face closer to the wall, making sure your arms stay as close to your sides as possible. That is, don't let them pop out like chicken wings. Bend only your elbows, keeping everything else in place, so that when you finish, your bent elbows will be right above the tops of your hips, as in Figure 8. Go slow! Keep your good alignment as you do the push-up. Be certain not to let your hips untuck, because this means you're going to put extra pressure on your lower back. If you need a reminder, look at Figure 4 again. Untucked

> Why are we doing push-ups in a book about legs? Because they teach you to have a connected core, which is vital to developing proper use of the lower half of your body.

hips also mean you are no longer connected between your hips and your shoulders, which means you're not exercising the muscles you should. To get the full motion, try to bend your arms until the tip of your nose touches the wall. Then come back up to your starting position. It's a small, controlled motion. Resist the urge to go too fast or fling yourself away from the wall. Remember, you're working on small support muscles.

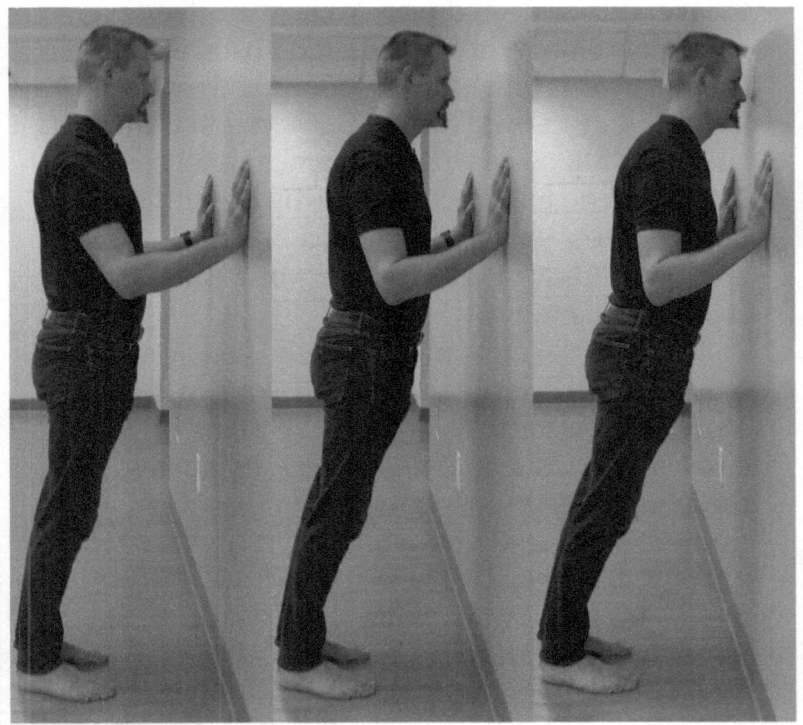

Figure 8: The range of a wall push-up.

Go try this now. Take this book with you and find a wall. Is your posture good? If not, feel free to imagine me shaking a stern finger at you.

...

Did you try it out? You'll get more out of this book if you experience what I'm saying.

Alright. I'm going to assume you did some wall push-ups, but I'm watching you.

Even if you have little to no arm strength, you should be able to do a few wall push-ups. On the other hand, if you are used to doing lots of push-ups or lifting weights, I'd still ask you to try this out and see what you feel. Go extremely slowly, holding a good posture all the way down. Hold for a count of one-one thousand at the wall. Then push yourself up to your starting position at the same (slow) speed. When you do a correct wall push-up, with good posture, you should start to feel some strain and little movements inside your shoulders around the joint.

These little movements mean you are not only using the large muscles of your arm, but also the little muscles around the joints of your elbows and your shoulders. Try to do ten of these wall push-ups three times a week, and you will quickly feel an improvement in the way your joints move. If that works, gradually increase the number you can do by three or four per session. Performing a lot of low-stress exercises will tire you out and thus improve your small muscles.

Try writing a reminder on a Post-it® and sticking it in an annoying place so you remember to practice.

Wall squats: while wall push-ups work on your elbows and your shoulders, this less intensive version of a squat will help you learn the small muscles around your hips and knees. In the upper body version of this, your shoulders are the ones benefiting most from improving the smaller muscles. In the lower body version, your knees will see the most benefit.

For this one, stand a little farther than one of your own foot's length away from a wall. You can check by placing one foot behind another to make sure you're out far enough. Lean back until your butt touches the wall. Again, using good posture—hips tucked, shoulders back, head back—slowly slide down the wall as far as you are able. If you are not used to squats, this may be only a few inches. If you are, it might be to where your thighs are horizontal to the floor, or even lower.

If you have not done squats a lot, I would advise only going down a few inches, certainly no further than where your thighs are horizontal.

The first time you try this, feel where your weight is in your feet. If it's mostly in your toes, then slide your feet out some. You want all the weight in your heels. You should *not* do squats where your weight is in your toes. That can cause injuries to your knee joints.

Once you are used to this exercise you can experiment with going down a few inches farther each time, until your butt is almost touching the floor. Remember to increment your squat *slowly*!

Alright, same drill. Take this book and go test it out. See what you feel. I'll wait here until you're done.

No cheating!

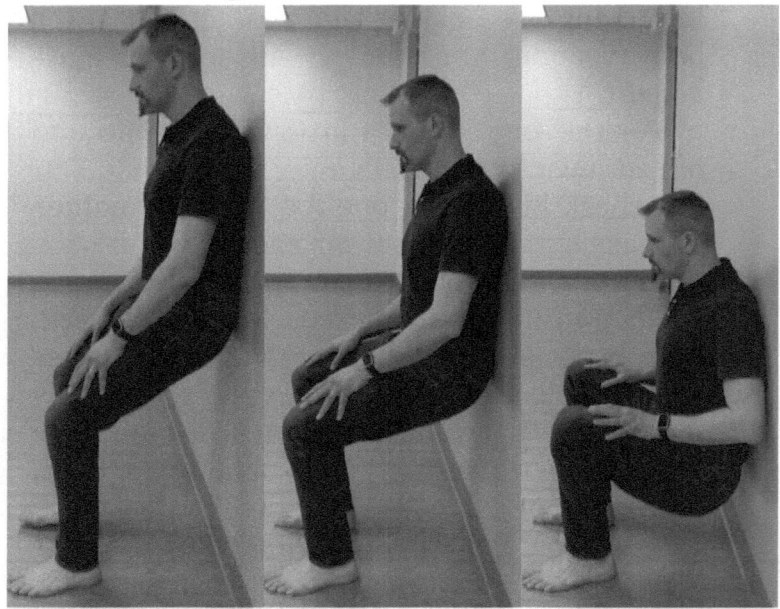

Figure 9: The range of a wall squat. Going past horizontal is the more advanced version.

If you do this in the correct posture, you should feel more stress on your knees and right above your knees than on your hips, simply because your hips are more used to bending while you walk. Did you feel all the little muscles activating around your knees? This is what you want to develop. With stronger support muscles surrounding your knee, you can resist your knee going the wrong direction if you step badly, or bending farther than it should. Squats also help your knees support more weight. Try to do ten of these three times a week and see what improvement you feel.

For both of these exercises, if you find them to be beneficial, slowly increase the number of repetitions over time until you get to twenty. For the push-ups, you can also step your feet further from the wall over time. For the squats, go a few inches further toward the floor over time. If you continue to do these exercises, you will strengthen your small muscles. They will then be able to help you out both in day-to-day motion and in strenuous exercising or bodybuilding.

Add wall squats to that annoying note you have pasted to your phone, your computer monitor, or your forehead.

Stretching

There is some debate on what you do when you stretch, whether you are increasing the flexibility of a tendon, or just the muscle, or some combination of the two. I'm not going to worry about that much here. Suffice to say if you stretch, you will increase your range of motion. However, it is possible to overstretch and damage something. It's as important to stretch the correct way as it is to stretch at all.

Stretching out your muscles allows you to operate your body to its full extent of motion. I usually do some amount of stretching every day, but if you'd rather have a more focused stretching session three or four times a week, that should be sufficient. You'll notice increased blood flow, better energy, and better flexibility by stretching regularly.

We'll be focusing on the whole body rather than just the legs, but it's important to stretch everything. Otherwise, the part not stretched will feel cramped up compared to the rest of your body. I know. I'm making you move around. It's awful. This is one of those things where you'll feel better after you do it.

How do you stretch? There are a couple different ways. One is simple static stretching. This is where you hold the position close to the extent of your range of motion for several seconds. Whichever muscle you are stretching may feel looser afterward and move a little easier. There is also dynamic stretching, where you move more quickly through the maximum and minimum range of motion of a joint, but don't hold the extents. Finally, there are a couple niche warm-ups and stretches called isometrics and pandiculation. Read on to learn about these fancy words!

At the end of this chapter, I'll give you the stretching sequence I teach to office-dwellers to keep them from hunching up like little toads at their computers.

Static stretching

Static stretching is the most common form of stretching and the easiest one to learn. Any place your joint naturally moves, you can go to the extent of that motion to stretch the muscle that connects to the joint. Some of the ones I like are shown below. Try them out one at a time while you go through the description. Some you can do while seated. Others you will have to stand for.

Neck stretch: standing in good posture (head, shoulders, hips, and knees—yes, I know I'm repeating myself. Are you still slumping?), turn your neck to the left to its full range of motion. Hold for a count of one-one thousand. For an added stretch, still in good posture, you can rotate your left shoulder behind you, also rotating your torso, which will give an added stretch. Then come back to a neutral position and go to the right. Next, lift your chin until it is pointing as far up as it can. Hold for one count. Then *relax* your neck downward, but be careful not to press your chin into your chest. Pressing down on your neck can cause damage. Last, you can stretch your neck side to side. Hold out your right hand and tilt your head to the left. This will lengthen the tendons in the right side of your neck. If you lower your

People often carry a lot of stress in their neck and shoulders. These stretches can help release that stress, or keep it from getting worse.

shoulder and pretend you are reaching for something you can't quite grasp, you will feel a nice stretch in the tendons and muscles that keep your head upright. Repeat with your left hand out and your neck tilted to the right.

Arm stretches: put both hands out in front of you, with one hand over top of the other. Extend as far as you can forward, then raise your arms as far as they go while your hands still touch. Then lower them as far as they go while your hands touch. Try to keep your shoulders relaxed as you do this. You can do the same exercise with your arms behind you, although this is more difficult. If you can clasp your hands together behind you, then do so and lift upward until you feel a stretch through your shoulder blades.

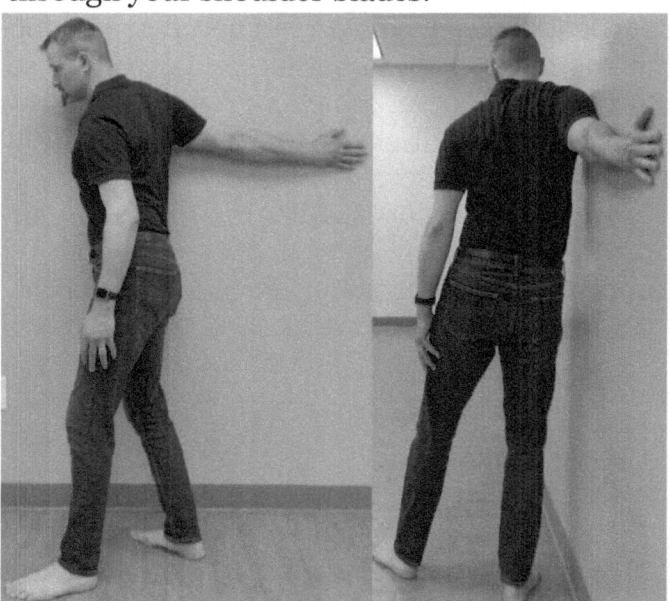

Figure 10: Arm and shoulder blade wall stretch.

If you cannot clasp your hands behind you, then stand next to a wall with one arm behind you and twist your body so your arm stretches in the same manner. Repeat on the other side.

Hip stretch: this one is easy. Simply stand in good posture, then lean your hip out to one side while keeping your head above your center. You should feel this stretch right below your hipbone on the side you're leaning toward. Hold for a few seconds then repeat on the other side. You can also get a good stretch to the back of your calf if you put the leg opposite to the hip you are stretching out by about a foot, rest on the heel, and lean back. If you need to, lean forward and put one hand above the knee of the leg extended for stability.

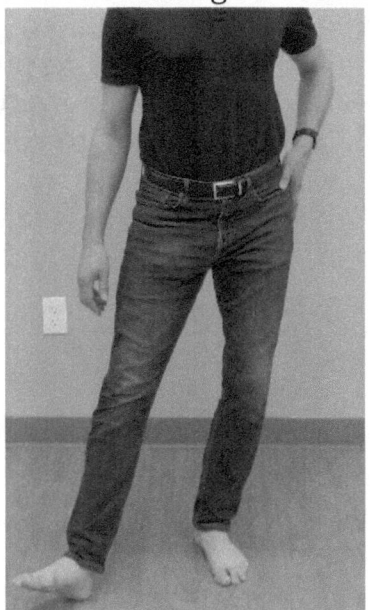

Figure 11: Hip stretch. You can also place your hand on your leg above the knee. You'll feel the stretch where the back hand is shown on the hip.

Leg stretches, part one: stand in good posture with your feet at hip width, then use your left leg to take a large step out to your left, with your left toes pointing 90 degrees out from your right toes (which you haven't moved). Turn your hips to the left so they are facing the direction you stepped out and bend your left leg. Try to lower your hips into the stretch, which you should feel mainly in your right leg. While you do this, make sure your left knee doesn't go beyond your left toes, as this will cause excess strain in your knee joint. If you look down, you should still be able to see your toes. Repeat on the other side. Try this same thing on both sides again, but after stepping out and turning your hips, also turn your back foot so it is facing the same direction as the front foot. Both feet will be 90 degrees from your original position. Try to press your back heel toward the floor, even if it does not touch, though make sure not to force it or hyperextend. Don't let your knee go past your front toes. This should give a good stretch along the back of your leg. Repeat on the other side.

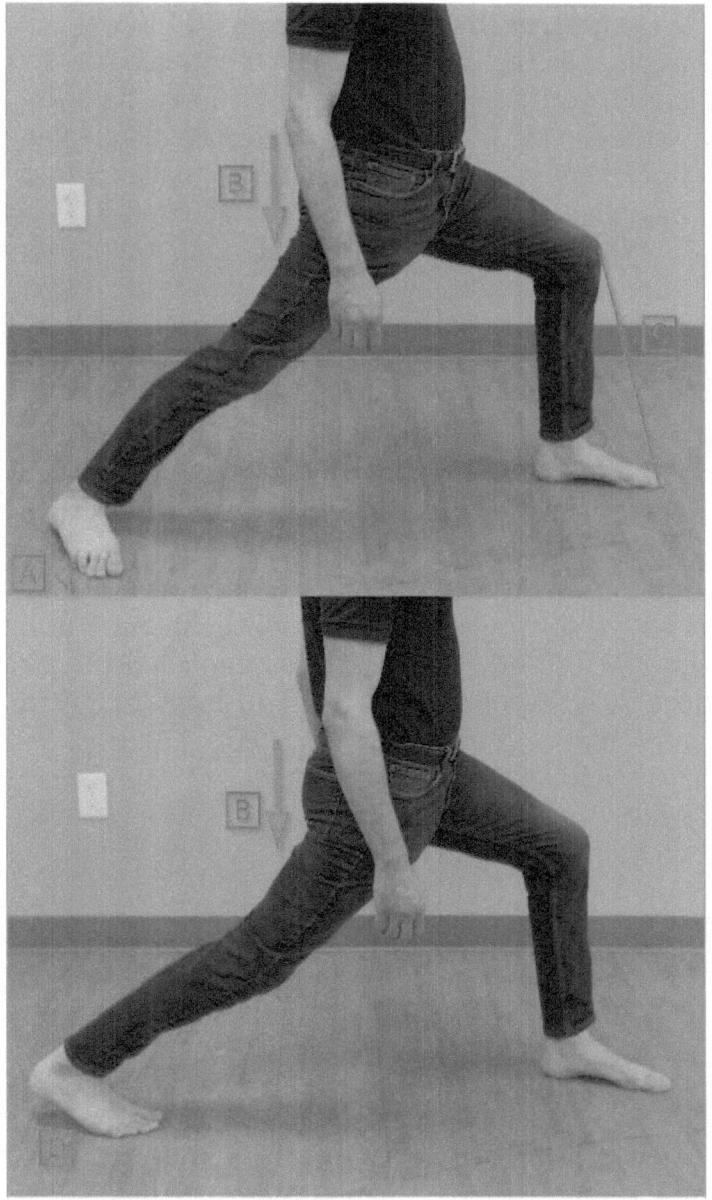

Figure 12: Leg stretches, with the rear foot pointed at 90 degrees (top picture, A) and straight (bottom picture). Sink your hips down in both stretches (B). Don't let your knee go over your foot (C). On the forward stretch, try to sink your rear heel down to the floor (D).

Leg stretches, part two: hold the wall, or a table, or the back of a chair if you need to for stability. This one requires a bit more balance. On the other hand, if you want more challenge, don't hold onto anything, and make this a balance exercise too. Just don't fall over!

While standing on one leg, pull the other knee up straight, as close as you can to your chest, holding with one hand. Count for about eight to ten seconds, then push your knee across your body for another eight to ten seconds, then to the outside for another eight to ten seconds. Next, let your knee drop until it points downward, and grasp your ankle with your hand. Pull your ankle up behind you. You should feel this stretch your quadriceps. Lastly (and this one takes even more balance and muscle, so don't worry if you can't hold it for long), hold your leg out straight in front of you and try to grab your toes with your hand. Make sure to bend your other knee while you do this for balance. Work on increasing the time you can hold each position until you get to twelve to fifteen seconds.

> Bend your knees and fight the robot menace! Flexing your support knee can give you a lot more balance.

Whew! That was a lot of work! Only one more stretch to go...

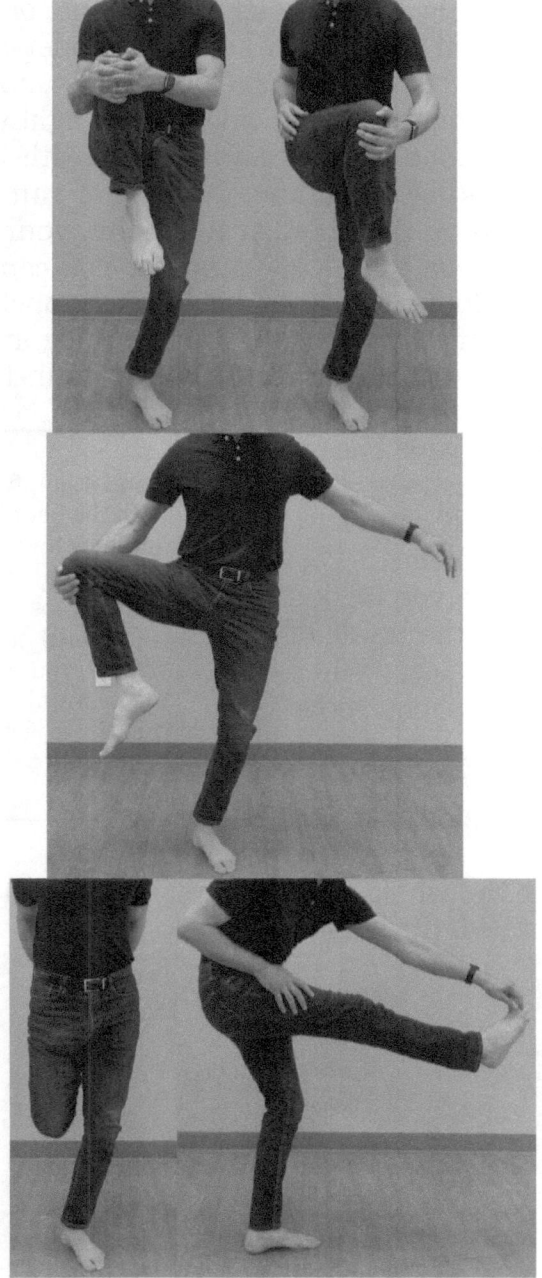

Figure 13: Stretching the leg up, in, out, back (or down), and forward.

Inner leg stretches: this is one of my favorite stretches, which I call the Spider-Man stretch. Start from a good posture (stand up straight!), then step out wide to your right with your right foot. Follow that leg down with your torso, bending your knee, until you can put your hand on the floor. At this point, your left leg should be completely straight. You can lift your left foot up so your heel is just touching the floor, if that helps. On your right leg, make sure your knee is directly above your toes, wherever they are pointed. If your knee is out of alignment with your toes, it can cause knee problems. This should give you a good stretch on the inside of your left leg. When you're finished, move your feet under you and raise your head and body slowly so you don't get lightheaded. Repeat the whole stretch stepping out wide to the left with the left foot.

> I find it helpful to turn both the bent knee and toes toward a 45-degree angle from the original position. And if you need more of a stretch, you can press the elbow of your arm into the side of your bent leg to push it out farther.

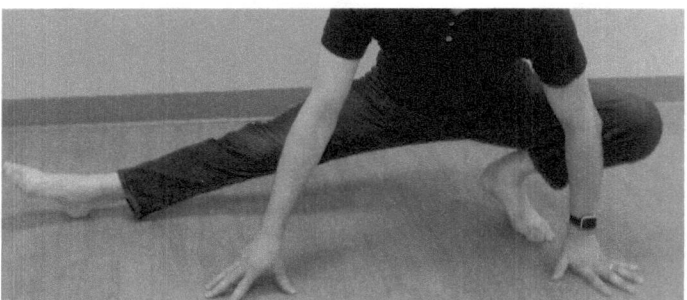

Figure 14: The "Spider-Man" stretch. Note the bent knee is in line with the toes.

This is a good introduction to static stretches, so let's go into dynamic stretches next.

Dynamic stretching

Dynamic stretching can produce a lot of the same results as static stretching, but in a shorter time. The drawback is that you must be careful not to hyperextend a joint (over stretch the joint in the direction it moves) while doing this. If you are double-jointed in your elbows or knees, pay special attention. It's best to start with a smaller range of motion and work up to the maximum range in which you feel comfortable. If it helps, keep a small amount of tension in the joints around the one you are stretching. If you've worked on the small muscles, this will be easier to do! For example, if you're moving your shoulder joint, keep your elbow a little tense so you don't flop around like a dead fish.

Here are some dynamic stretches I like.

Neck stretches: the neck is fairly susceptible to injury, so be careful when you do this. Don't go past your range of motion and don't jerk your neck. First, as in the static stretch above, tilt your neck to one side (bringing your ear closer to your shoulder), then tilt to the other side. Stop for a moment when you get to your range of motion before going back to the other side so you don't strain your neck muscles. You can also look straight up, then bring your chin down to your left or right shoulder, then straight back up, then down to the other shoulder. These two stretches together should cover the range of motion of your neck.

Arm stretches: First make sure you have enough space around you. That's a whole arm's length in front, in back, side to side, and above you. Watch for hanging lights, kids, cats, and knick-knacks on tables!

Now, swing your arms forward, starting slow and moving a little faster if there's no pain or resistance. Reach all the way above your head when you do this. Full range of motion! Try to make your fingers touch in front of your face, then separate as they pass your waist. Make seven to ten circles.

This is another of my favorites, especially when standing up from sitting a long time, usually in front of a computer. When you type, you tend to keep the rest of your body rigid and your shoulders don't move.

Next, reverse and swing both arms backward so your arms are coming up from hips to shoulders, then around in back of you. Try to touch your fingers as they rise in the front, and keep your arms close to your head as they go around. Don't strain your shoulders to reach too far behind you. Also do this seven to ten times. After you get used to this maybe go up to fifteen revolutions, but you don't need to do more than that.

Your arms should be feeling nice and loose at this point. Now you want to move your arms through their horizontal range of motion. Start with your arms extended straight out away from your sides, then come forward with both until your arms cross and your hands are hugging your opposite shoulder. Reverse direction and swing your arms behind you through their full range of motion, touching your hands together behind you if you can. If it helps to find your range of motion, try to clap your hands together in front and touch your fingers behind you. If you have a large range of motion, you may be able to clap behind your back as well! Repeat this about ten times or so to really loosen the shoulder joints.

Torso stretches: while keeping your pants button or belt buckle facing forward, try to turn your shoulders from left to right and right to left. You should feel a line of tension reaching from shoulder to hip when you do so. This exercise can help to loosen up your lower back as well. Repeat about seven or eight times. You can twist a little harder on this one as you generally won't overextend anything here.

Hip stretches: This one is very nice for loosening your pelvis. Start from—what am I going to say? Yes, from a good standing posture—then bend forward so you can touch the ground with your fingers. If you can't touch the ground, move your feet out to a wider stance. Bend your knees for more balance. Then with your hands on your hips, circle your upper body, leaning to the left, behind you, to the right, and back to the front. Take a very brief pause in the front. Repeat five times, then switch and rotate the other direction. As your hips become more limber, you will be able to circle your torso at a deeper angle.

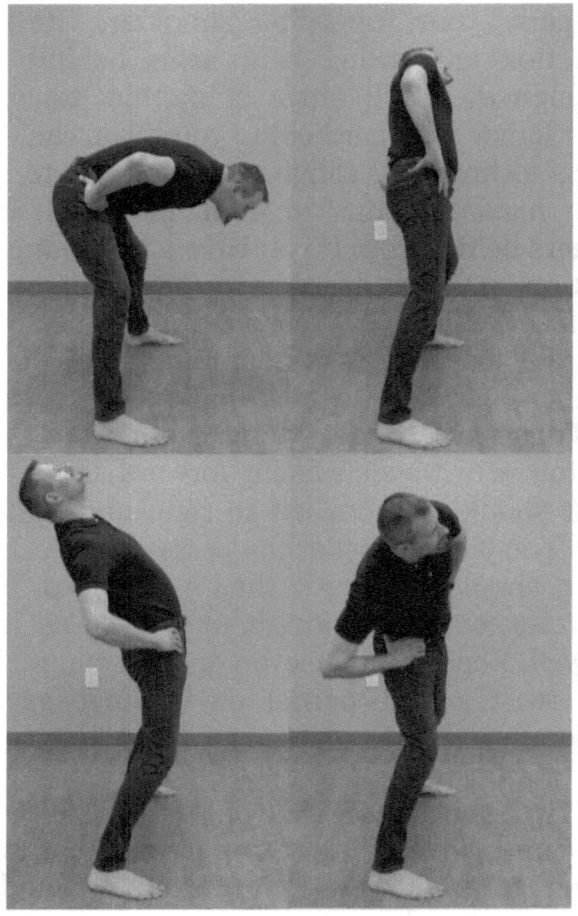

Figure 15: Hip stretches, moving circularly around the waist.

Leg stretches: this one is very easy in theory, but make sure you don't lift your leg too high and strain your hamstring. Use control and don't let the momentum of your swing determine how far your leg goes. Hold on to a chair, table, or wall if your balance is not the best. Start from a good posture (as always), feet under your hips, then swing one leg as far as it will go up in front of your face. Let your leg come back down with gravity to touch the floor with your toes about one and a half feet (half a meter) behind your starting position. Repeat eight to ten times with each leg. Try to engage your quadriceps and hamstrings when you do this, so you are pushing and pulling your leg up and down, rather than just swinging.

Knee stretches: bend at the hip and knees by about ten degrees and place your hands on your knees. Rotate your knees in small, slow circles, about the width of your foot. Your knees are not able to bend very far to the sides, but this circular motion will open up the joint. Repeat eight to ten times, both clockwise and counterclockwise. If you really want to, you can also do that move where you switch your hands over your knees, like your weird uncle does.

Ankle stretches: stand on one leg, making sure to bend your support knee (grab something for balance if needed!), and trace a circle about one and a half times the length of your foot with the toes of your raised foot. Go both clockwise and counterclockwise ten to twelve times. Stand on the other leg and repeat with the opposite foot. As an added bonus for this exercise, you can pair your hand motion to get a dynamic wrist stretch. While you have one foot in the air, trace a circle in the air with your fingers about one and a half times the length of your hand while you do the same with your foot. Go both directions with your foot and hand moving at the same speed. For an added *added* twist that will really break your brain, try going clockwise with your hand and counter-clockwise with your foot, then vice versa! This one is good for flexibility, balance, and coordination.

> There are a lot more variations of dynamic stretching that you can experiment with. Just make sure you don't overextend your joints when you try them out. And remember that good posture! I bet you've already forgotten.

Isometrics

Isometrics is the act of tightening your muscles without changing their length, both to warm up and to increase your flexibility. I'll give you a few exercises both for your arms and your legs, but you can also come up with others on your own. If you've never done this before, you may get a warm or buzzing feeling in the muscles you do this with. That's normal, and not, in fact, angry bees trying to escape your flesh.

Leg stretches: to demonstrate how this works, we'll do the easiest version first. Start from a good posture—head back, shoulders back, hips tucked—and bend your knees slightly with your feet about the width of your shoulders, or a little bit wider. Plant your feet firmly on the floor, and starting with your thigh, pull inward with your entire leg, as if you want your feet to come together. But don't let up the downward pressure on the floor! Your feet should stay in the same place. Tense your knee joint to protect it so it doesn't bend (like we did in the dynamic stretches), and try to pull your legs together with a fair bit of force.

Your legs may shake, and you may feel them grow warm. Still not bees. Hold this stance for a count of ten-one thousand. Now reverse, and while holding the same stance, keeping the muscles around your knees tense (which are more developed now you're doing squats, right?), push your feet apart, starting from the thighs. Again, your feet should not actually move. This time you'll feel the muscles on the outside of your legs engage and perhaps grow warm. Hold this for about ten seconds as well.

Come back to your good posture, this time with your feet about hip width apart, so narrower than before. Take a big step forward with one foot so your front knee is bent, and your back knee is mostly straight, though not locked out. Just as last time, tighten your muscles around your knees and don't let your feet or legs move. Then pull in as if you want both feet to slide directly under you. You'll feel the same stretch and warming sensation, this time on the fronts and backs of your thighs. Reverse this and push your front foot forward and back foot backward as if you are doing a split (but don't really do a split).

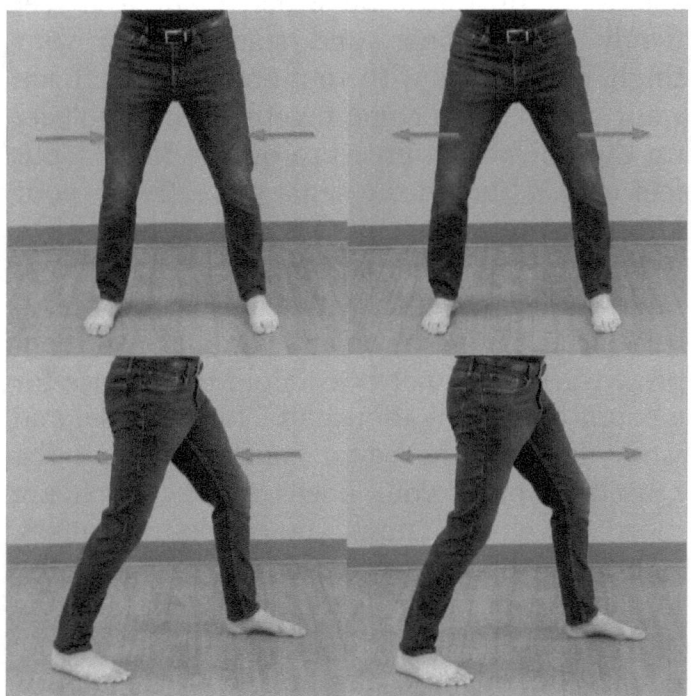

Figure 16: Isometrics, pulling in and pushing out standing with legs parallel (top) and after stepping forward (bottom). The force starts from the thighs.

Hold each position for about ten seconds. Next switch your legs so the other one is forward, and repeat both the pull in and the push out for about ten seconds. After this, your legs should be nice and warm, and your muscles should feel engaged.

Arm stretches: Let's try the same sort of exercises with your arms. You'll either press together as much as you can or pull away as much as you can. Here's the setup for your arms: put your hands together palm to palm with your fingers turned 90 degrees so you can clasp your hands together. Have your elbows bent a little bit more than 90 degrees and push your hands together. Keep your shoulders down while you do this, because otherwise you can put too much stress on your shoulder joint. Then reverse and try to pull your hands away from each other while they're still clasped together. You may want to lower your arms a little bit to make sure your shoulders are not raising up. Hold both of these exercises for about ten seconds.

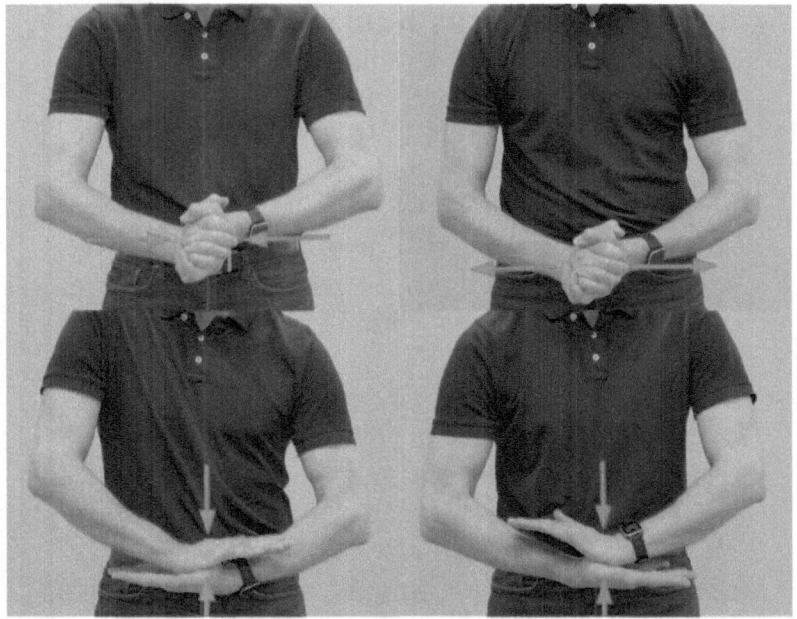

Figure 17: Isometrics, pushing in and pulling out (top) and pressing down with either hand (bottom).

For another variation, hold one hand just under your bellybutton, palm up, and close to your stomach, as if you're holding something up. Now put your other hand on top of the first one so the heels of both hands touch, and press both hands together. Don't let the muscles around your elbows and shoulders move, similar to what you did with your knees for the leg stretches. Keep your hands at about the level of your bellybutton while you do this. Remember to keep your shoulders low! Switch hands and do the same with the other hand on the bottom.

Those two exercises (pulling horizontally, then vertically) tend to get my arms feeling limbered up and warm. If you want some variations on this, you can put your palms and fingers together as in the first exercise, but this time keep your hands aligned so your fingers touch. With your fingers pointing upward, you can press your hands together and move slightly upward from your chest to about your chin, while pressing inward. Switch your hands so your fingers point down, you can do the same thing, pushing your arms inward, while moving from around your bellybutton to your hips. This one tends to work your chest muscles a little bit more, as well as the stabilization muscles in your shoulders.

Isometrics can be a great way to warm up when you're doing weight training, or if you're about to do hard exercise. These are also very nice if you've been sitting at a desk all day and your shoulders and legs are stiff. They can create the same effect as stretching out, but in a much smaller space.

Pandiculation!

Pandiculation is a fancy term for the involuntary stretching of the soft tissues, which you do while yawning. You know where you put both arms up above your head and sort of tense at the same time you reach your arms as far as they go? That's pandiculation. It's similar to the isometrics I talked about above, but rather than using two limbs in opposition to each other, you're tensing individual limbs. The exact feeling is hard to describe, but it's sort of like pulling inward at the same time you're pushing outward.

> Pandiculation acts as a way to reset your neuromuscular system, especially if you've held the same position for a long time. If you've seen a cat or dog stretch after taking a nap, this is pandiculation.

It works as a kind of neural feedback loop to adjust how much tension you have in your muscles and put them back where they should be. Afterward, you may feel your shoulders, for example, falling into a relaxed position, especially if they've been up by your ears all day from dealing with stress. Because it's never easy to move when you're all tense, pandiculation also works to get you ready for activity.

Try it out yourself. Think about yawning, or read about yawning, or even just say yawning a lot. Yawning. Are you yawning yet? When you yawn, stretch your arms above your head and let them do what comes naturally. Do you feel the pandiculation function? If I'm sitting down, I like to continue the motion after stretching upward by putting my hands on my thighs and pressing downward. You can activate the same pandiculation response, and I find it often opens up my shoulders a lot (you might hear some pops and cracks!). Afterward, your arms will probably feel looser, as if you've just stretched them out.

You can do the same motion with your legs, for example if you stand up after sitting for a long time. Stand up and let the pandiculation response take over (yes, I like typing that word). I feel a tightening going from my knees, up through my upper thighs and into my butt. It feels similar to the isometric exercise where you're pulling your legs in toward each other. Afterward, continue the feeling by reversing direction and pushing out and down through your feet.

Feel out the involuntary response that happens. Then learn how to channel it so if you feel stiff, you can pandiculate on command! But don't overdo it, as this function is still partially involuntary. You can mess up your joints if you do it too much or try to tense too much.

Observe when this happens naturally. Try to mimic the function voluntarily in your arms, or legs, or neck, or hips. This is similar to how I teach a lot of my martial arts classes. You can only teach somebody so much when breaking concepts down to their fundamental principles. At a certain point, you have to teach a person to observe themselves while they do an action, then let them copy and expand upon what they observe.

Add pandiculation to your stretching toolbox. The reason I give you so many types of stretches is because different stretches work better for different people. Try them all out and see what gives you the most benefit.

Stretching sequence

You can find a video of this stretching sequence at: youtu.be/aniANeMQYio

This is a sample of the stretching class I used to run at my day job once a week. This is geared for people who work primarily in an office, often sitting down for long periods hunched over a computer. There are a couple challenges if you're not used to complex motion or standing on one foot. If you do work in a desk-bound or sedentary job, this sequence of stretching may help you out as well. You don't have to restrict yourself to once a week either. If you do this every day you'll see a definite increase in your flexibility, and potentially a reduction in your tension or knots in your shoulders and back. Even running through this sequence two to three times a week will help. I usually go from the head down to the feet because it flows well for me. You don't have to do this, and can go from feet to head, or even just whatever feels best at the time. But try this stretching sequence as it's written a couple times to get used to it and see if it works for you. You'll notice this combines elements from both the static and dynamic stretching sequences, plus a couple extras.

Posture first! Fix your head, shoulders, hips, knees, and feet. I haven't harped on this in a while, but you should be used to doing it. You have been practicing, right? Using a timer to remind yourself? I'll assume you said yes. It's hard to hear through space and time.

Wrist stretch: This is good to loosen up your wrists if you've been using the computer and mouse for a while. You may hear a lot of popping and cracking in your wrists! First put your hands together, palm to palm, and press down and away from you to stretch your wrists (see the top two pictures in figure 18). Your elbows will pop out from your sides, and you can wobble your hands back and forth to open your wrists up. Do this for about five seconds. Then switch so the backs of your hands are together, with your fingers pointing straight down. This time pull your arms upward and slightly away from your chest to stretch the other side of your wrists. Hold this for another five seconds, rolling the backs of your hands across each other.

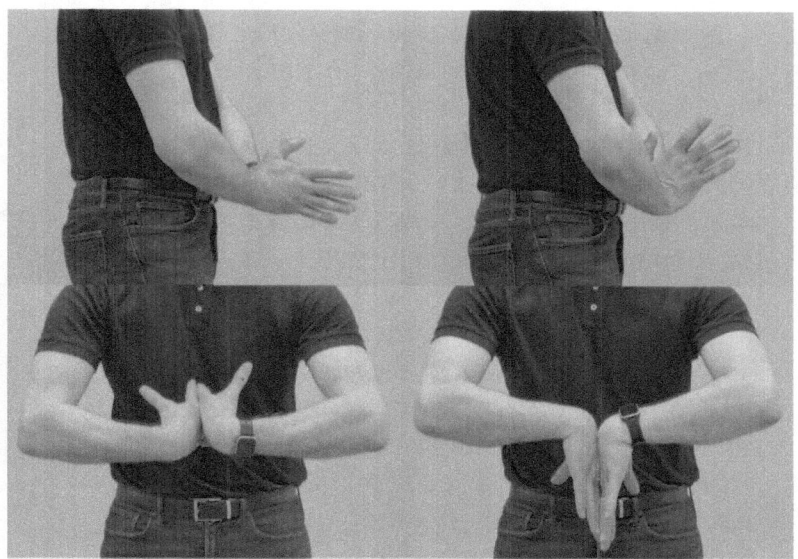

Figure 18: Wrist stretches with palms together (top) and backs of hands together (bottom).

Wrist, elbow, and shoulder rotations:
Next, roll your wrists in circles through their full range of motion for eight to ten rotations. I like to go clockwise with my right hand and counterclockwise with my left to start so my hands are moving "outward." Then switch directions and roll the opposite way ("inward") for another eight to ten rotations. Keep your fingers loose while you do this. Now relax your wrists and move the rotation up to your elbows. Go outward and then inward in the same way, eight to ten rotations. Last, do the dynamic shoulder stretches described above, making big circles, using your full range of motion. Go forward, backward, then across your body. Make sure you have enough room and don't hit any furniture (or pets), including behind you!

Neck and torso stretches: Get into your good posture, and expand upward as if your head is connected to the ceiling on a string, and the string is tightening. While looking horizontal (that is, don't look down or up), turn your head as far as it goes to the left. Hold this for a couple seconds, then turn your shoulders to the left as well, while making sure your knees are still in alignment with your toes. Hold for a few more seconds and feel the diagonal tension across your chest. Then repeat this sequence while looking to the right.

Next, continue with the static neck stretches described above, by looking up, then down. You can include some dynamic motion when you look up, by turning your chin side to side. Finally, do the static neck tilt, first to the left and then to the right, each for about ten seconds. Remember to reach your arm out to the side as if you can't quite reach something and drop your shoulders to get a good stretch in your neck tendons.

Torso twist: This is the same as the dynamic stretch above. Just keep your belly button facing forward and twist your shoulders until you feel a diagonal line of tension from shoulder to hip. Twist in both directions five to seven times.

Lower back stretch:

This is a really good static stretch for opening your lower back, particularly if it aches. Simply lean forward and let your arms dangle to the floor. Your knees should be slightly bent. If you need to spread your legs out to touch the floor, that's fine. If your fingers are dangling in the air, that's fine too. What you want to focus on is letting the lower vertebrae in your spine release. Feel how, when you're bent over, your back slowly releases with the pull of gravity, since it's now going the opposite direction of how it's usually positioned (good upright posture, right?). The important part is to relax. If you're very stiff, or if you have a known back injury, your back may hurt while you bend over. Try to feel where it hurts and see if relaxing that area lets you get closer to the floor. I'm talking here about "stiff" hurting, not sharp pains or continuous pain from injuries you know about. If you have a hard time relaxing, read through the next section, then come back to this one!

A warning on this one: if this hurts a lot, don't do it! There may be something else wrong you need to get checked out. If you have a known back issue, clear this stretch with your doctor first.

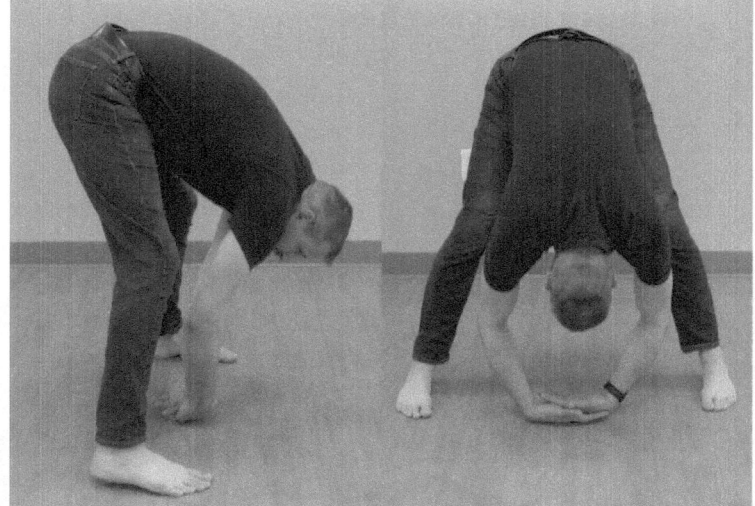

Figure 19: Lower back stretch. Make sure to relax into this position slowly over at least fifteen or twenty seconds.

During this stretch, you should feel your spine lengthening, and your hands will gradually get closer to the floor. If you need more distance, bring your feet in some to let you stretch further. Hold this...well, really, hold it as long as you want. This is a position that benefits from the feedback of learning how to relax while you do it, which then lets you relax more, which then gives more feedback, and so on. Whenever you're done, come up SLOWLY. You've just sent a lot of blood to your head while leaning over and if you come up too quickly, you may get tunnel vision or even fall over. It's best to "roll" up as if your back is a garage door that's opening up vertebrae by vertebrae until you're vertical (and in good posture!) once more.

Hip stretches: This is a good time to do the dynamic hip rotations from the previous section to loosen the connection between your upper and lower halves shown in Figure 15. Do five in each direction.

Leg stretches: From here on out, everything is about legs. The sequence I like to do is as follows. First do the static leg stretches, part one, from above (Figure 12: stepping out to the sides, first with your feet at 90 degree angles, then with your feet in line to the left and right). Then do the static hip stretch (Figure 11), including putting your foot out in front for the foot raise and calf stretch. For a quick ankle stretch, get in good posture, and rock up to the balls of your feet, then back on your heels. Put your hands out in front if you need to, to keep your balance. Go from toes to heels seven or eight times.

Next do part two of the static leg stretches (Figure 13), lifting one foot at a time to stretch out your quadriceps and hamstrings. As an added ankle stretch, you can rotate the foot that's in the air around in circles, both clockwise and counterclockwise. If you feel really adventurous, add in

Remember to use a chair, counter, or table for stability if you need to. These exercises give you a great chance to work on your balance!

hand rotations along with the foot rotations. If you go different directions with your hand and foot, it'll break your brain!

As an alternative, if you don't have a lot of time for leg stretches and do have a lot of space, you can do the dynamic leg raises to stretch both the quadriceps and hamstrings. Just be careful not to go too far and overextend, and also try not to kick anyone walking by...

Finally, do the static inner leg stretch, or "Spider-man" stretch (Figure 14). Come back to the center after you do both sides and roll up again as you did for the lower back stretch.

Shake everything out. You'll feel nice and relaxed, and probably energized. Once you get used to this sequence, you should be able to do it in ten minutes or so. Doing it twice or three times a week will help your balance, flexibility, and coordination.

Remember, you're getting used to new muscle configurations. If you haven't done these types of stretches before, take it slow and let your body get used to it. Getting a massage or having a hot shower are good ways of getting tension out of your muscles while adjusting to more efficient movement.

Relaxing

We've talked about stretching out, but you should be able to relax, too. The biggest enemy of moving efficiently, or even using your body at all, is tense muscles. If you've ever seen professional fighters, or a gymnast, or a highly talented musician preparing to play, you may notice it looks like they're doing things effortlessly. That's because they are relaxed. They aren't fighting their own body.

An action—surprise!—is easier when your muscles aren't opposing that action. When you learn a skill and have repeated it so many times that it is innate, you "relax into it." You do this because you are not frightened or uncertain about what you're going to do. You've got this. It's easy.

Remember when you first learned to drive a car? Or if you don't drive, ride a bicycle? Or if you don't ride a bicycle, any other skill that takes a lot of time to master? The first time you do it, you're very tense, you're very uncertain, you don't know if it's going to go right in the end. You tense up. This makes it harder for you to learn as you don't know what you are doing, *and* you have to fight against your own muscles at the same time.

If you are tense in everyday motion, you add the energy required to tense your muscles to the amount of energy needed to perform that action. Let's reverse that trend. Your ideal state is to be completely relaxed when you're not actively doing something requiring muscles to engage. When you do need to use your muscles, there are some other tricks to give you an advantage. I'll cover some of those at the end of the book.

For right now, we're going to focus on simple relaxation. As before, let's start from the top. Stand, or sit, or lay down. It doesn't really matter where you are. Actively focus on the top of your head. There are a lot of little muscles you don't think about that cover your skull. Now's the time to pay attention to them! The first challenge is to *be aware* that you can change the state of these muscles. When you're focusing on the top of your head, work to relax everything there. When it works, you'll feel a shift as the energy you're unconsciously holding in these muscles leaves, and they slide back to wherever gravity puts them.

After the top of your head, go down to your ears, and particularly your jaw. Pay attention to where your jaw meets the bottom of

> Many people, especially when they are stressed, put a lot of tension into their jaw muscles.

your ear all the way down to the bottom of your chin. Relax this whole system. Let the tension drain out. You may feel your jaw hanging open slightly. Often you just need someone to call attention to the tense area to realize it is tense. In fact, this area gets so tight that you can take another "pass" along it and relax more muscles the second time. Do this as many times as you need to feel all the tension in your jaw drain away. Once you lose the top layer of tension, you may feel another place you can relax, or you may immediately tense up again because your body is so used to doing so. Persuade your muscles it's alright to relax completely.

Your jaw is tied into your neck muscles, which are then tied into your shoulder muscles. The jaw is a huge lever that needs to be strong enough to tear through tough food. Thus, it's hinged nearly at the centerline of your skull. You may not realize it, but everything from your shoulders up to the top of your head is affected as you chew. So, if you are artificially keeping more tension in your jawline, that stress is reflected back into your neck, your shoulders, and your head. This is why you may get a headache when you're tensing your jaw. It's also why you may grind your teeth when you sleep while stressed.

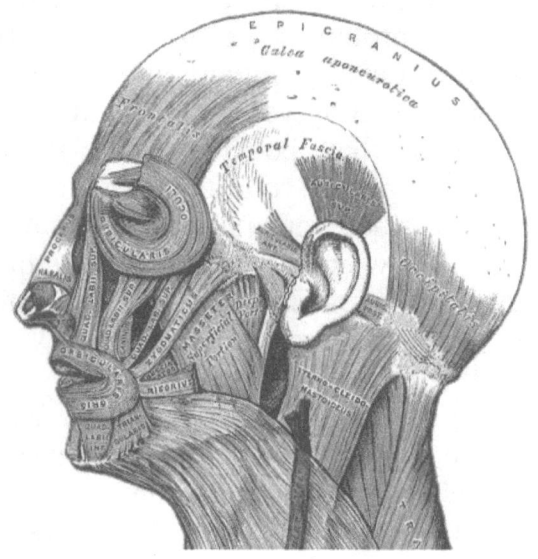

Figure 20: There are a lot of muscles to relax in the head (*Gray's Anatomy*)!

Relax these muscles. I bet they've gotten tense again while you've been reading about tense muscles. I know mine have. This is often the first thing I notice if I am under pressure at my day job or have a deadline coming up. This is another good place to set a timer. This one might be as short as five seconds! Depending on how you deal with stress, you may clench your jaw tightly without even realizing it. In order to develop the habit of *not* tensing it, you must be aware of what's happening.

Now your jaw is relaxed (is it still relaxed?), let's keep moving down your body. Next is the shoulders. Remember the exercise from the beginning of the book? Up, back, and down. Or if you realize you're raising your shoulders up, simply let them fall. If you have your shoulders relaxed, it's a lot harder to tense up your back. Many back problems come from this combination of tense shoulders and tense jaw, because you're holding your upper body weird and—remember that bowling ball? If that weight is right above your center where it's supposed to be, then your back doesn't have to contort into a new shape to hold it upright. If you're hunched forward, tense, and tightening your jaw, you're making your back deal with a load extending forward.

Relaxing your lower back is another really good exercise, which I talked about last section in the stretching sequence. Now you're more aware of how to target individual muscles, try that stretch again and really pay attention to the muscles along your spine and in your lower back. Spend as much time as it takes to stretch out. If I do this, I'll basically end with my forearms horizontal and my elbows touching the floor after a bit of stretching.

The rest of your body tends to fall into line after you relax these parts. However, the other two areas that may be a problem are hands and feet. Remember to take breaks while you work to stretch them out. A really nice one is the wrist stretching exercise I detailed above in the stretching sequence, Figure 18.

Especially if you do manual labor, or are on your feet a lot, your extremities can get tired, then try to compensate for the tiredness by tensing up.

Next, rotate your hands around the wrist in little circles. Switch and go the other direction too (this is also similar to the stretching sequence above). Curl your fingers in, then spread them wide. Repeat. Especially if you've been typing on a computer, you may hear a lot of little crackles in your wrists and hands as they open up.

You can also massage your hands. Hold your left hand out, palm up. Support the back of that hand with the fingers of your right hand. Now you can press your right thumb into the palm of the left hand. Especially concentrate on the pad below your thumb, and the web between your thumb and forefinger. Press—as hard as you're comfortable with—between the bones of your fingers, and also on the meaty pad below your pinky. Switch hands and do the same for the other one.

Obviously, this is hard to do with your feet, especially if you're wearing shoes, but the same actions apply. I can tell you, it feels really good to push a thumb right in the middle of your foot. You don't often get that feeling, especially if you wear shoes a lot.

Is your jaw tense again? How about your shoulders? I'm not being condescending here. This is also a reminder for me.

> Note for author: good posture, relax your jaw, untense your shoulders. (edit: ahhhhhhh.)

Add another note to the timer you set to maintain your good posture. You have done that, haven't you? When it goes off, reset your posture, then remember to relax as well.

Connection (Not the opposite of relaxing!)

The concept of connection is intertwined with relaxing, but is not the same thing, nor is it the opposite. To illustrate what I mean, let's use your hand as an example.

I like to think of your body as having three levels of tension. The first is completely relaxed. Hold your arm out and completely relax your hand. You may have to work at this because you're used to holding some tension in your hand. If it's completely relaxed is going to flop over the air and dangle from your wrist. If you shake your arm your fingers will wobble around. This is completely relaxed, which is not actually very useful, unless you're lying down. If you completely relax your body, you collapse into a pile of limbs.

On the opposite end of the scale is complete tension. Don't do this for long, because it's not good for your joints and can cause cramps, but if you fully tense all the muscles in your hand, your hand is going to curl into a claw. Also, not very useful, unless you're controlling the motion and turn your hand into a fist instead. This requires some other body mechanics, and a little bit of martial arts knowledge, so I'm not going to go into that here. For this example, and for general daily usage, you don't want to be fully tensed.

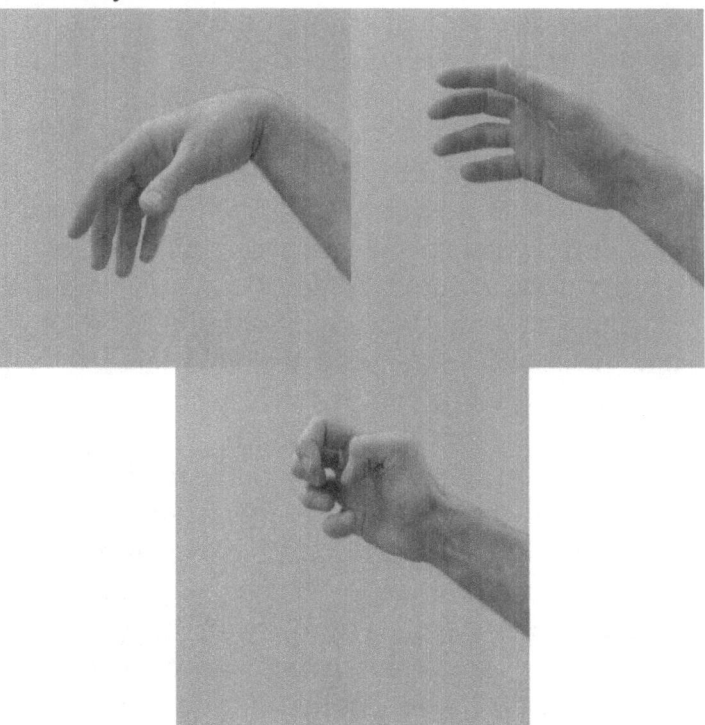

Figure 21: The hand fully relaxed, with connection, and fully tensed.

Last is what I like to call good connection. You use this a lot of the time, without realizing it. This is what you do when you are standing up but not doing any activity. What I want to teach you is to use the same good connection throughout all of your body rather than just portions. So for your hand, if you put your arm out in front of you, just holding your hand out "neutrally" is using a good connection in your hand. You're not letting it completely collapse, and you're not turning your hand into a claw. When you have a good connection, you can still move your fingers around and rotate your wrist, but there's just enough muscle usage to resist gravity. If you concentrate, you can feel a little tension to resist your hand fully collapsing. Now we're going to apply this concept to the rest of your body.

Again, get in your good posture. Head, shoulders, hips, knees. You will naturally be using a good connection for your legs, and if you put your hips and your shoulders in the right position, you should feel this tension in your abs as well. If you use a "lazy" posture as I described in the first chapter, with your shoulders slumped and your butt sticking out, this relaxes the muscles in the front of your body. That means you don't have to maintain a good connection with your abs, but your abs surround what? That's right, your center. So, it's beneficial to always have good connection in this part of your body. If you center is engaged, then you connect your hips to your shoulders, and it helps you stand or sit up straight.

Get in your good posture again (because you've probably slumped out of it while you've been reading, right?). The act of pulling your shoulders back and tucking your hips underneath you puts your abs in alignment. It should be easy to start feeling a good connection. If you can still relax your belly and let your stomach come out, try this: stretch your head up as if it suspended on wire. When you do this you're going to "expand" your body upward, and it is going to be very hard to keep your stomach relaxed. The reason I'm focusing on abs is because this is the main muscle that connects the lower half of your body—your legs—with the upper half of your body—your arms and head.

Let's try again. This time, relax, then put a hand on your belly. Loosen your abs. Now, while holding your hand on your stomach so you can feel the changes, get into a good posture. Feel how this affects your abs. Now expand upward, stretching so you feel your head connected to the ceiling by a wire. When you do this, your abs should stretch out even more and you'll be forced to maintain a good connection between your hips and your shoulders. While keeping everything else in place, just try to relax your abs. It's pretty hard!

Here's one last quick exercise to show you why keeping a good connection in your abs is helpful. First, we'll do the relaxed situation. Shake out your body and go back to your regular stance, whether your shoulders are rounded, butt is out or whatever. Twist your shoulders from side to side, then bend to your left and bend to your right. Your hips don't have to move while you do this, do they?

One last time (for right now), get in a good position, tuck your hips as in Figure 4, and expand upward. Feel the connection of your abs between your hips and your shoulders. Now do the same exercise: twist your shoulders and try to bend to your left and right. You should feel your hips start to come along with the motion. This is because you've now connected your hips to your shoulders, and that is what I mean by connection rather than relaxation.

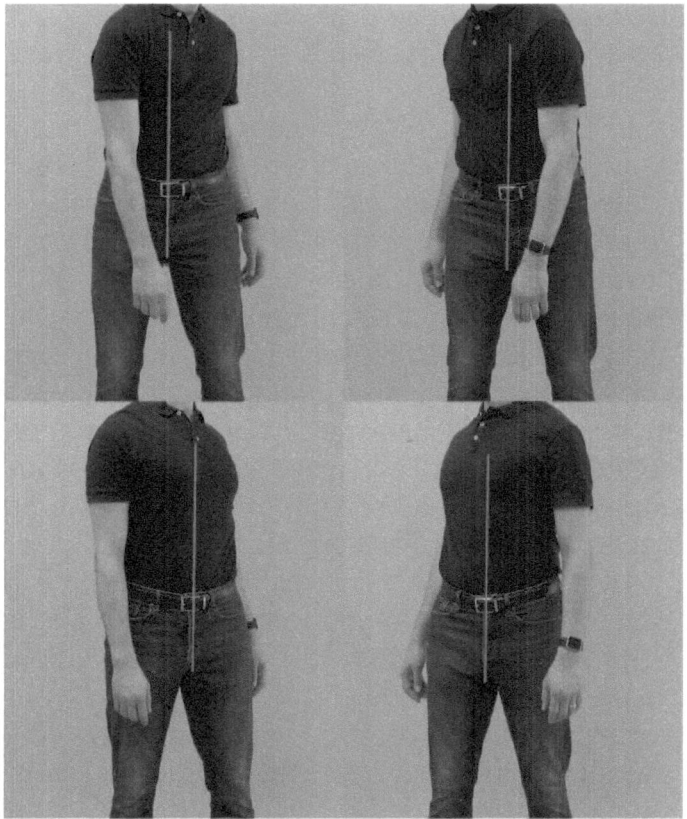

Figure 22: Note the hips don't move when twisting with little connection. With good posture and connection, the hips start turning with the motion.

Remember how this feels, because after we go over some basic leg anatomy, we're going to put all these concepts together into the main idea of the book: how to walk. But, we're coming at this from first principles, as if you're completely new to this body you have. You (hopefully) understand by now how to keep yourself limber and relaxed, with good posture. Now, rather than learning to crawl before walking, we're learning how the body is connected before walking.

Anatomy of the Legs

This next section details the anatomy from your feet up to your core. I won't be naming muscles (mostly), but I will be going through some of the kinematic connections and how your lower limbs are supposed to work. Please don't skip this part. Paying attention to how your body is connected is one of the major steps in learning how to operate it. I promise I'll make this as exciting as possible.

Why are we only looking at anatomy up to your core? Because this book is subtitled "The Legs," even though I've been covering the entire body to this point. That will now change...

Feet and Ankles

I bet you think about your hands a lot, since you use them every day for all sorts of activities. However, how often do you think about your feet in the same way? They are equivalent to your hands in many respects, although you put more weight on them, and they are specialized for the action of walking rather than grasping and manipulating. That said, they can still do a lot of the same things, and you can use your hands as an example of how to learn to operate your feet better. For this section, if you have the freedom to, take off any shoes and socks, and let your bare feet contact the floor. This will help you feel what I'm talking about.

We'll cover more on this topic at the end of the book where we review the action of walking, but for now, place your feet flush to the floor, then try to feel where your foot contacts the ground. If you have flat arches, this may be nearly the entirety of the bottom of your foot. If you have regular or high arches, your foot may only contact along a "C" shape going from the pads of your feet to your heel. Then there are those stubby things at the end of your feet. What are toes for anyway? They don't have the same manipulative power as your fingers do, but they still play a big part in your balance.

Move your feet through their whole range of motion. Stand on one foot, lift the other up, waggle your toes, and roll your ankle around as in the leg section of the stretching sequence I covered in the previous section. You have a bunch of joints in your foot—just as many as you do in your hand. These can be incredibly helpful if you use them while you walk. They also help you balance. Stand up

Can you lift your toes up while you leave the rest of your foot on the ground? Can you move your toes individually? If not, it's likely because you've never practiced. This is why it's important to explore your anatomy (and yes, I know how that sounds...). You may be able to do things you never thought you could, just because you've never tried.

straight with good posture (as usual) and try to move your balance around with just your feet. Can you push off with your toes so much that you start to tip backward? Can you pull with your toes and go forward? Rock up to the balls of your feet and back to your heels as in the stretching section, but this time, feel how your toes react.

There's another axis of rotation for your feet which people often disregard, and that is side to side. Try rolling to the outsides of your feet so you're just standing on the "ridge edge" of your foot. Let your knees push outward as well, so they are still above your feet. If you can hold this position, you may find that it's actually more stable for balance than standing flat on your feet. Ha ha! I've tricked you into something I'm only going to explain in more detail at the very end of the book. Now you're going to have to keep reading!

For now, let's move on to the next joint.

The Achilles Tendon

The Achilles tendon is vital to walking. We found it before, in the section on muscles, tendons, and ligaments at the beginning of the book. I hope yours is still in the same place.

I'll give you one really good exercise for your Achilles tendon. This also has the added benefit of helping to prevent plantar fasciitis, which is the inflammation of the strip of connective tissue on the bottom of your feet between your heel and your toes.

This one is pretty easy. Just stand with good posture and bring your center slightly forward so that it's over your toes rather than over your heels. As you do this, you will naturally start to raise your heels, just like the exercises with your center from the first chapter. Use this motion, with your weight over your toes, and push upward, extending. Hold for about five seconds, then put your heels back on the ground. You can exercise your Achilles tendon by doing these heel raises. It's easy to do while you're standing somewhere, for instance brushing your teeth. Just come up to your toes and then back down to the ground. You can also find a ledge (for example, a stair close to ground level) so that rather than coming back to ground you can flex until your heels are lower than your toes. Be certain of your balance and don't fall! This will give an added dimension to help stretch out the fascia on the bottom of your foot. You'll also feel this lengthen your Achilles tendon and exercise your calf muscle.

If you stand for long periods of time, or your Achilles tendon is tight, or weak, then you run the risk of inflaming the plantar fascia (that connective strip). Moving your feet around, wiggling your toes, and rolling side to side will help.

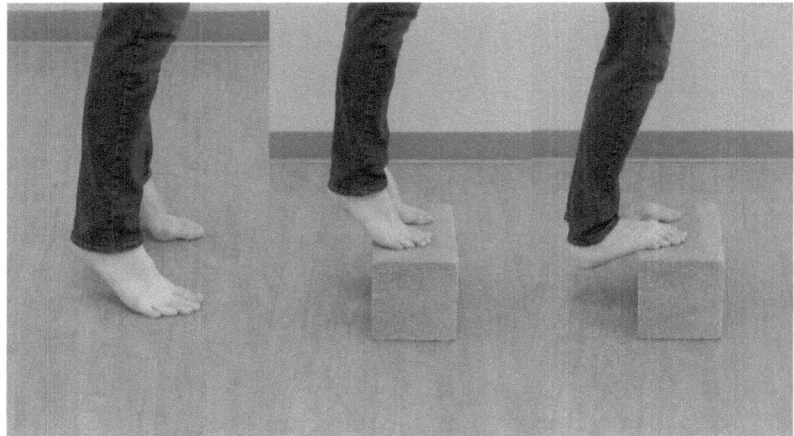

Figure 23: Calf raises on the floor (left) and on a ledge (right).

See if you can hold this stretch for a few seconds before you come back down. As you get better, try to extend the total time you can stand on your toes. Try for ten seconds. If you can do that, then go for longer. If you do this every day, add a second or two each time you do it. Soon you will be able to stand on your toes for longer periods of time. This is also really useful if you're trying to reach something up on a high shelf!

As a final challenge, once you get proficient at this, come up to standing on your toes and the pads of your feet only. Hold this. Walk around on your toes. If you are used to high heels, this may be pretty easy. If you're not, this is a great calf-building exercise. Plus, it's just cool to do.

Your Knees

Let's talk about your knees. Specifically, the relationship between your knees and toes. I often get on my martial arts students about this, because if you bend your knees wrong a lot, you can mess up the knee joint over time. Then you're due for a knee replacement later in life, which is a big hassle and a lot of pain. Avoiding it with proper posture and movement is easier, less painful, and will save you a lot of money.

First sit down in a chair. Remember your good posture! Your shoulders should be back, your head above your center, and your feet out in front of you. In this position, your knees should be directly above the center of your feet. This is generally where you want to have them whatever you're doing. Now stand up. Again, your knees should be above your feet. This is the orientation you should keep for almost everything you do.

Try this exercise briefly while standing, but don't leave your knees in this position: Keep your feet steady on the floor, toes pointing straight forward, but start bringing your knees in as if you are going to make them touch. Do you feel that stretch or strain in the outside of your legs? You may also feel some tension on the side of your knee facing your other leg. Go back to your starting position, knees over toes. Do the same thing but outward. If you push your knees outward, then you should feel the opposite strain on the inside of your calf and on the side of your knee facing out from your body. Come back to center. If you try to put your knees in these positions while you do any sort of activity, that tightness that you felt will be magnified, and can lead to straining or rupturing ligaments or tendons. This is what happens if you step wrong and roll your ankle, for example.

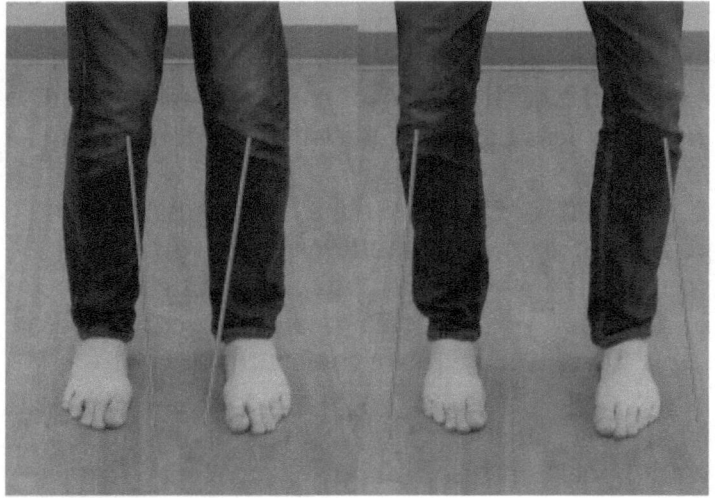

Figure 24: Your knees should line up with your toes. Here the knees are not lined up, causing excess stress.

If your knees aren't straight, the weight on your feet is not going straight up (or down) your leg. Instead, it's going to the side of your leg, away from the powerful muscles in the middle and into the smaller, more fragile supporting muscles on the outsides of your knees. If you are holding a heavy object or doing some activity, the load on your feet can go up by a significant fraction of your body weight.

When you walk, you should not let your knees drift to the inside or the outside of your feet. Even if you bend your knees, or squat down, your knees should stay in line with your toes.

Note your feet can rotate quite a bit! Your knees should follow them. So if, while standing, you turn your toes in toward each other, your knees should be facing inward, right above them. The same thing should happen if you turn your feet out forty-five degrees, so you make a large pizza wedge. Your knees should also now be pointing out forty-five degrees to each side—above your feet. If your knees don't follow your toes, you'll get the same stress as described above, and potentially cause damage to the knee joint.

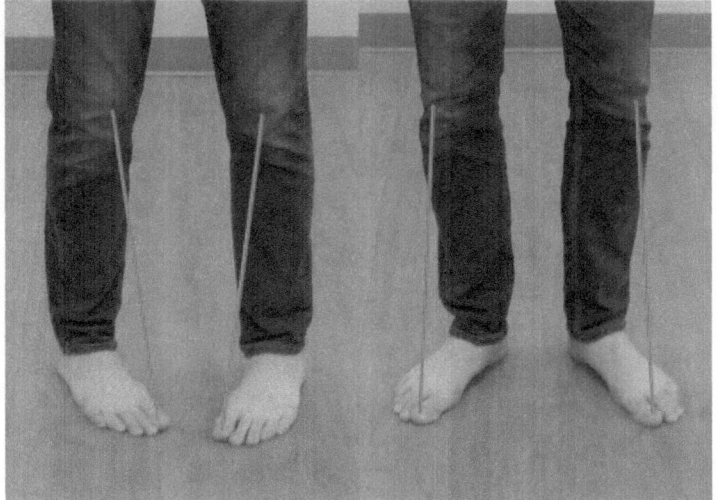

Figure 25: Here the knees are aligned with the toes.

Knees and elbows—whose connective roles are similar—are two of the joints that take the most abuse in daily action. An exercise to help combat degradation and injury in your knees is squats. Often the subject is met with a groan as it's not popular like bench presses or leg lifts, but I'm going to spend some time talking about them because they're very important for good leg health.

Let's go through the process of a good squat. I described a squat on a wall in the muscles section. If you've mastered that, this is the next step. First, get in a good posture with your feet about your shoulder or hip-width apart. Second, I want you to start the motion with (surprise!) your hips. Because they're tucked under you (they are tucked under you, aren't they?), you can reverse that and start to stick your butt out. If you did the example showing how to move your center, then you know you'll feel like you're starting to fall backward. This is what you want to feel in this instance. You can put your arms out in front of you to help with the change in your center of mass. Try to get your center over your heels rather than over the center of your feet. This is going to force you to work on the correct muscles for a good squat.

Your eventual goal is to get your butt almost to the floor, but it's perfectly fine to start with squatting only a few degrees, then slowly increase your squat until you get your thighs horizontal. If you need to, hold onto a tabletop or counter with your hands while you do this to make sure you don't fall backwards.

Start bending your knees more and more, making sure to keep them over your feet, and don't let them drift to either side. Go down as far as you are able, keeping your hands out in front to help your balance. You should feel like you're almost falling backward the whole way down. Keep your torso upright, and don't give into the urge to lean forward—that will put your weight over your toes, which will both defeat the purpose of the squat and put your knees under more stress. Come back up, slowly in the same manner, still with an upright torso. Finish in a good posture.

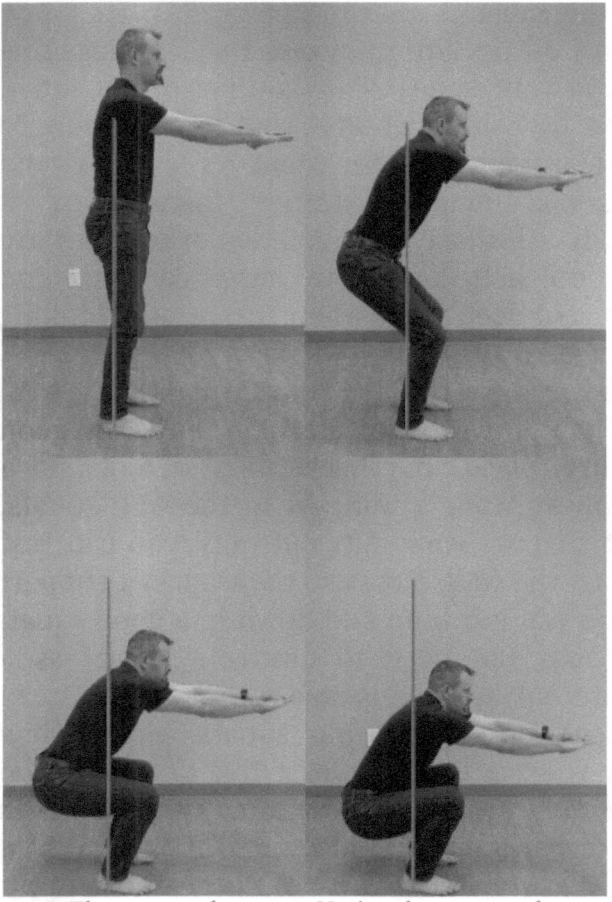

Figure 26: The stages of a squat. Notice the center of mass (red line) stays above the heels.

If you're keeping your weight on your heels, you might have to step back and catch yourself sometimes. This is fine! After getting used to going down to where your thighs are horizontal (as shown in the lower left in Figure 26), work your way down until you can just about sit on the floor.

Do the squat very slowly for best effect. Once you understand your balance while moving, try it without holding on to anything. You'll use your leg muscles more!

Feel all the little muscles that are engaging around your knees while you perform a squat. These little muscles are what you're going to build if you do the squat in a slow and controlled manner, rather than doing it quickly. All those little muscles, when they are built up, help keep your knees centered and over your feet, even when you're not thinking about it.

If you have trouble doing squats, here's an alternate way to get started. While in good posture, place your heels about a foot and a half away from a wall. As in the wall squats, start sticking your butt out until you can rest against the wall. Now use the wall as a support so you can move up and down in a good squat. You may not need to use your hands as a counterbalance in this case.

However you do your squats, making it a daily routine to do at least five or ten can be incredibly beneficial in building up your knees over a period of a month or so. If you want a challenge, try to work up to thirty squats every day, and do it over a month. You can also change up how deep your squats are. See if you can get your butt all the way to the ground, then back up to full standing position. As you get better at this you can move your feet closer together to give you even more of a challenge.

> The key to squats is to start small. The best starting place is probably the squats with your back against the wall, just to make sure you don't injure your knees, which is the whole point of this. Try to do ten of those a day for a week and see if your knees feel stronger. Keep either adding more squats or going lower slowly and steadily, and you'll be surprised what you can do!

Thighs

Your quadriceps (in the front of your leg) and hamstrings (back of leg) are the equivalent of your biceps (top of your arm) and triceps (bottom of arm) in your upper body. But the muscles in your legs are generally much larger than the ones in your arms. They are the powerhouse of your body, along with your core muscles. The squats I described above will help you develop these muscles, along with the small stabilization muscles around your knees.

But while your quadriceps and hamstrings are very powerful, is always important to look at the connections at the ends of the muscles. A powerful crane is only as good as the foundation it's built on. If you can lift 100 pounds (or 45 kg for you metric types), but the connection between your quadriceps and your knee can only support 90 pounds (fewer kg...) then what happens? Your crane crushes its base. Except instead of a base, it's your knees. Muscles usually connect near a joint, and joint problems are one of the hardest things to repair or heal.

Let's look at the end of your thighs near the knees first. They are one of your most exposed joints, along with your elbows. Take a seat and let's go through some of the muscle connections. Put a hand on your knee and let your fingers trace where the tendons join to the kneecap. We're going to go through those connections, then to their other end, where the tendons disappear into the large muscle of your quadriceps.

Keep your hand on your knee and slowly stand up from where you're seated. You should feel the muscles on the sides of your knees retract, or move out of the way, while the tendon connecting the top of your kneecap to your quadriceps gets very tense, then relaxes when you fully stand up. There are a whole bunch of little connections here, and if any one of them gets damaged, the rest of them have to take over to

> I find the motion of the kneecap one of the most interesting in the body. Your mileage may vary.

help. The more you can protect and strengthen these tendons the better.

Let's try this again with the underside of your knee. Sit back down, then put both hands on one of your knees so that your thumbs are on the top of your leg and your fingers wrap around underneath your knee. You should feel several large ropey tendons on the underside of your leg connecting your lower leg to your upper leg. If you explore very carefully, you should feel two on the inside and one on the outside. Sit all the way straight back in a good posture. Now, while lightly gripping your leg, I want you to stand up. Feel those tendons shift around? If, for example you're feeling your right knee, and you lean very slightly to your left as you stand, you may feel the tendons on the interior of the underside jerk before you stand up. These are the tendons of your hamstrings activating to pull your body forward so that you can stand. You can feel the same sort of thing if you stand on one leg (with a bent knee), and open and close the leg that you have in the air with your hand underneath your knee. You'll feel those tendons go taut, then relax.

This is sort of like the hinge of your leg. You know those metal doohickies on the top of screen doors? When you open the door, they extend and slowly retract back to close the door. This is a similar action to what's going on with the tendons underneath your knee. They provide a lot of explosive power to your movement, especially with things like running or jumping.

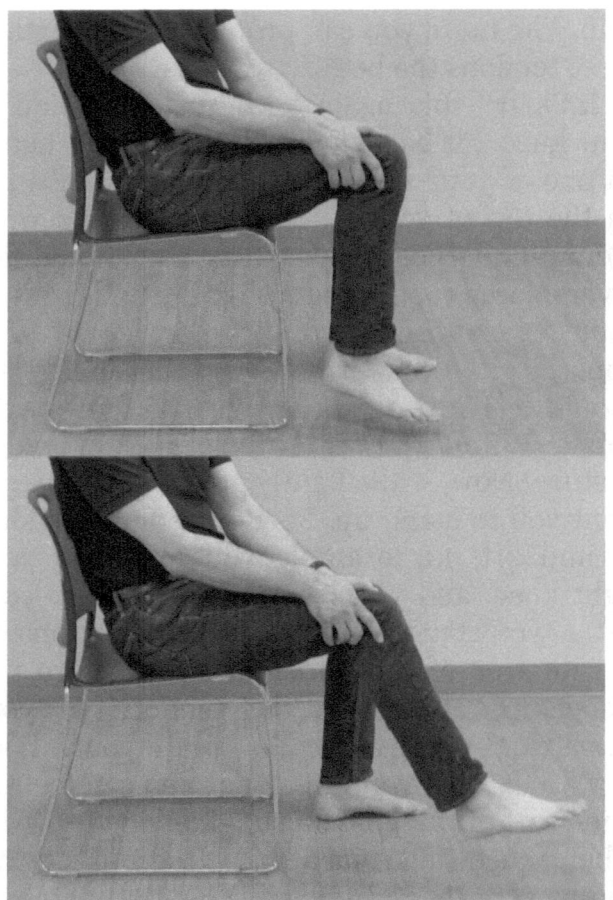

Figure 27: Feel the tendons under your knee to better understand how your thigh muscles work.

Now, since you're feeling yourself up, move your hand through the lower portion of your thigh, even to that ridge underneath your butt. Try the same exercise: sitting down and standing up while feeling this area. You may need to use both hands because this muscle is much larger than your knee. Along with the major contraction and expansion of muscles you may also feel something like hard ridges that suddenly pop up, then disappear, especially on the inside fold between your quadriceps and your belly. This is similar to what's happening in your knee. You're feeling the tendons go rigid in order to pull your muscles quickly to a new position. This, in turn, pulls your bones where you want them to be.

There are a lot of little stabilization muscles around the joint of your hip and if they weaken, or if any of them tear, then the rest have to take over for them. That increases the wear on the hip joint, and you're on the road to eventual hip replacement!

Okay, now that we've talked about the ends of your thigh muscles, let's talk about the muscles themselves. First, the quadriceps (the ones in the front of your leg). These muscles act in opposition to your hamstrings, just like your biceps and triceps act in opposition to each other. This enables you to move your leg (or your arm) in very quick motion because you can pull on both sides of the bone in quick succession, thus moving it very fast. The quadriceps is the muscle group that has four "heads" reaching all around your kneecap. The other end attaches up into your pelvic bone. You can feel this if you put your finger right where your hip bends, then lean over a little bit. You'll feel a hollow appear as the muscle contracts and expands.

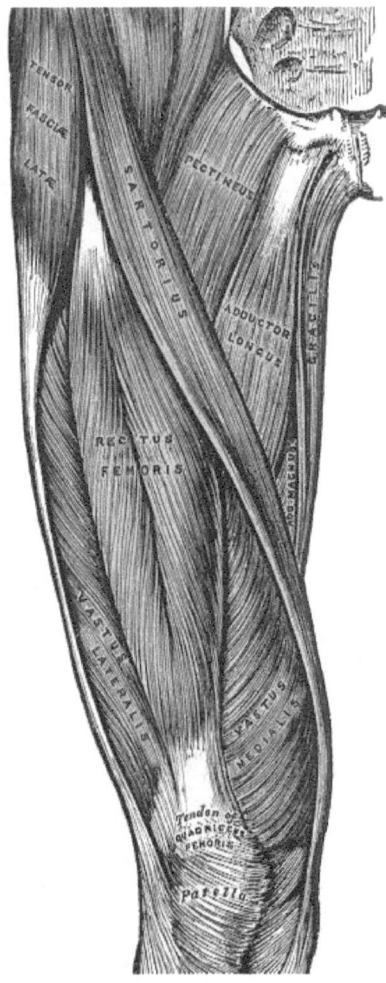

Figure 28: The muscles of the thigh (Gray's Anatomy).

Interestingly, the large head of the quad that makes up that impressive bulge on gymnasts, swimmers, and other athletes (the rectus femoris, seen in Figure 28), is actually pretty weak in helping you stand up and in extending your knee. The other three heads of the muscle do more, because they connect to the sides of your knee and help stabilize the entire compound muscle on the front of your thigh.

The hamstrings work in opposition to the quadriceps, but only some of the time. Try this exercise: put one hand on the front of your thigh (the quadriceps) and the other hand on underside of your thigh (the hamstring). Do the same exercise of going from a standing position (in good posture, right?) to a seated position.

You can feel how both muscles pull on your leg bones while they support your body in motion. However, they activate at different times with the quadriceps working a little harder while you sit down and the hamstrings working a little harder when you stand back up. You can also feel a difference while walking. Put your hands one on top and one on bottom of your thigh again, then take a step with the *opposite* foot. You'll feel the quadriceps relax a little bit as the other foot goes forward and the hamstrings tighten. Then as you pull that foot forward to take the next step, you'll feel the quadriceps start the movement. This pushing and pulling motion is the majority of how we walk and is tied directly to your hips. You didn't think I'd forgotten about your hips, did you? We'll learn more about this push/pull motion at the end of the book, but for now, let's move onward and upward. Even though this book is called "the legs," we can't round out the topic without talking about how your legs connect to the rest of your body.

Hips

The hips. I can talk about these joints for a long time. I've taught several martial arts classes focusing almost exclusively on the hips and how they move. They are the equivalent of your shoulders for your lower body, but unlike your shoulders, they support your weight all the time. Thus, for things like posture, lower back support, walking, and even sitting at a computer, your hips are very important, and you shouldn't forget about them.

Let's try a similar exercise to the one in the previous section. Put your hands on your hips with your palm right on the edge of your pelvic ridge (which should be the thing holding your pants up on the left and right of your waist), your thumb going forward around the circumference of your hips, and your fingers trailing down into where your quadriceps meets your butt. Now walk.

I've been talking about the hip area for the whole book. Yes really. Go back and look if you don't believe me. Posture: tuck your hips. Center of mass: this is where your hips are. Stretching: contains both a static and dynamic hip stretch. Hopefully you're starting to realize how important these joints are. It's what joins your legs to the reason you have legs.

Okay, wait, come back. Did you remember your posture? Fix it.

And take this book with you.

Okay, now walk.

The first time, walk about ten steps with your hips in the "lazy" position, with your belt buckle pointing downward. Then turn around and walk back to where you started. Next walk back and forth with your hips tucked like I told you in the section on posture. You feel all those little connections and moving tendons and muscles in your hips? These are all the connections that keep you upright, and let you walk. And...I actually can't go into this in as much detail as I want right now, because I haven't taught you how to walk yet!

Even though you are most of the way through this book, we haven't gotten to the really juicy bits yet. For now, remember how all those little connections felt underneath your hands. Go for a long walk and just feel how all the little muscles wrap around your hips and activate as you move your legs. Stand still and shift your hips around in a little circle. See which muscles activate while you do that. A lot of this you're going to have to feel for yourself. Keep in mind what I've gone over with your quadriceps, hamstrings, and hips. There will be a test later.

Glutes

You knew this was coming, didn't you? You're going to feel your own butt. Put one hand on each of those glorious glutes and take another walk. You can leave the book here for this one. Just remember your posture and keep your head up and your hips tucked. Make this walk a little bit longer. Try to walk around objects, or turn corners, or lean forward and backward.

Go on, I'll wait here.

Are you back? Did you feel all the connections and the different muscles activating as you moved? Obviously, a lot of this overlaps with your hips, since they are connected to your butt. Different parts of your glutes trigger as you take steps and move in different directions. Keep these connections in mind when I teach you how to walk. For now, I'll give you an overview of the structure of your gluteus. Think of this as Hips: Part Two. Again, the reason we're talking about this in a book about your legs is this is the all-important area of connection between your lower and upper half.

Your butt is made up of three main muscles: the gluteus maximus, medius, and minimus. Most of what you feel is in the maximus muscle. In contrast, some of the upper connections when you were feeling your hips was the gluteus medius. Most of the minimus is hidden underneath the medius, and like the little stabilization muscles in your knees and shoulders, mostly helps you keep your hips level as you walk. The whole gluteus collection of muscles is specific to humans because we are the only animals who walk completely upright. It can help you stand up for long periods of time, especially if you use good posture. Were you wondering if I was going to bring posture up again?

While the gluteus muscles help you stand up, if you sit down for long periods of time—for example if you are in an office job—the gluteus can weaken. You want to make sure you take care of it. One good method is the squats I described near the beginning of the book, and again in the section on your thighs. Try a squat with your hands on your butt and see how the muscles change shape!

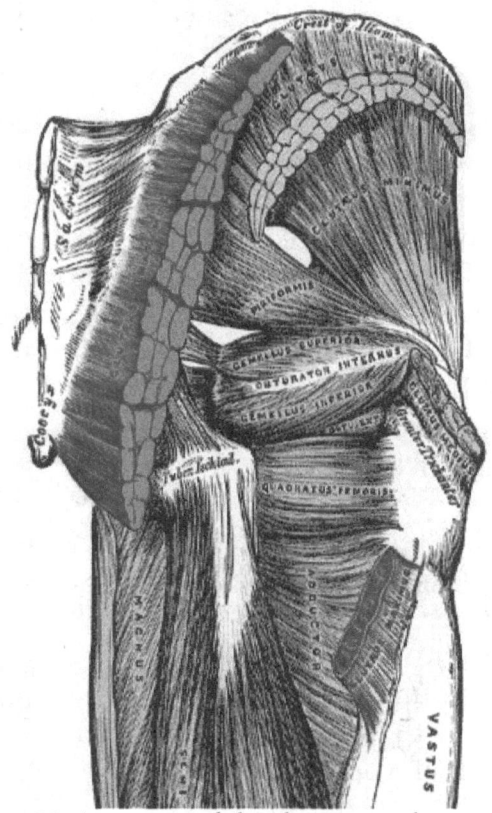

Figure 29: A cutaway of the gluteus muscle group (Gray's Anatomy). The maximus is cut away (highlighted), as is the medius.

Without such strong muscles keeping us upright, we would start to bend forward like an animal walking on all fours. Now you've got a little experience holding on to your butt as you walk, you'll be able to feel the difference when you walk efficiently rather than walking, well, like you usually do. Stay tuned!

Core

This section of your body could probably have its own book. As your hips are the connection between your lower and upper half, your core contains the muscle that lets you activate it. By no coincidence, this is also where your center of mass resides. Remember how I said if you control the center of mass of something, you control how it moves? Your core muscles can help make the difference in graceful, efficient movement, and lazy, slow movement.

Another concept many fitness guides don't cover is that the muscles in your back are just as important as the ones in your abdomen. If you've got really developed abs, but haven't worked on any of the musculature of your lower back,

Why are we talking about these muscles in a book called "the legs?" Because this is the highest area of the body where musculature connects directly from the legs. Your core is also connected to your arms and head, so it overlaps nearly all musculature systems in your body.

you're more likely to slump forward, and also more likely to have lower back problems. We'll briefly go over the anatomy of your core muscles as well as those in your lower back.

First the big one—what people call the abs. If you do a good crunch, or bend forward, you will feel three "stopping" points in your abdomen.

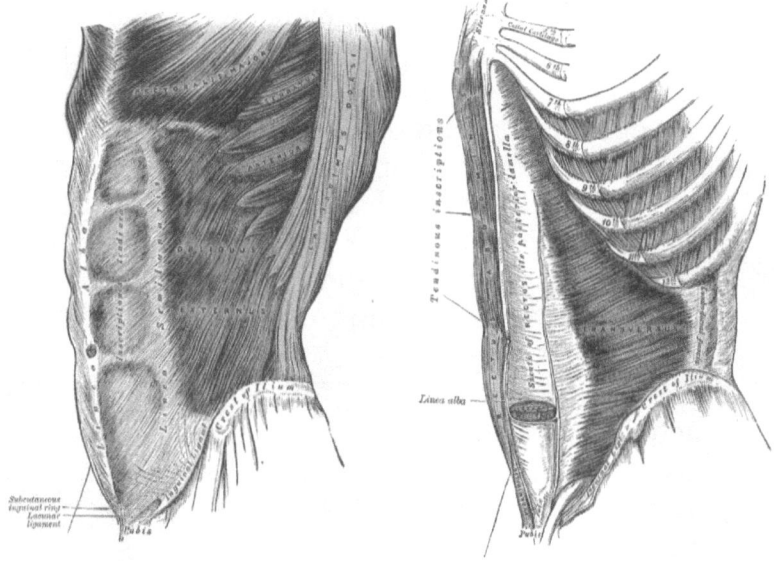

Figure 30: The muscles of the torso, notably showing the rectus abdominis and the bundles of musculature (Gray's Anatomy).

Just as we did with the other sections of your body, put one or both hands on your abs while you bend over and see if you can feel how this area moves. This is all one giant muscle, divided up into multiple sections. Officially, it's called the rectus abdominis, and no, that's not the name of a dinosaur from a *Jurassic Park* movie. This paired muscle (one on each side of your bellybutton) goes all the way past your sternum—that little nubbin in the middle of your chest—down to your groin. The reason it feels like a lot of small muscles (and why we call it a "6-pack" when you can see it on someone) is because there is a bunch of connective tissue between parts of the muscle. The "packs" are bundles of muscles, like a handful of straws. The connective tissue is the same stuff tendons and ligaments are made of, but they're not called that because neither end connects to bone.

So what? This band of muscle is the primary way we flex our spine forward. It connects your ribs to your pelvis and keeps most of your internal organs inside your body. It's also used in maintaining that semi-relaxed connection I spoke about above. When you stand up straight and expand upward, like you've been practicing this entire book (you have been practicing, haven't you?), this band of muscle engages from groin to rib cage. It's the largest area in your body that doesn't have a solid internal structure.

Although your abs keep your rib cage from flopping forward over your hips, they don't actually connect your upper body with your

The only bones inside your lower torso are your vertebrae, which are only a few inches or centimeters around, and are in the back of your body. What's holding up all those juicy organs? This band of muscle. Along with your hips, I would say this is one of the most important areas of your body to pay attention to in everyday action.

lower body. There's only one muscle that does connect all the way from your spine to your leg bones, and that is the psoas (pronounced "soaz") major. This is an internal muscle, but it's the muscle that lets you pick your leg up while you're standing upright. Get in your good posture, then lift your knees up in front of you like you're marching. You're using your psoas major to do this work. If you march in place for a while, you'll start to feel a burn around the center of your leg. This is where the psoas connects.

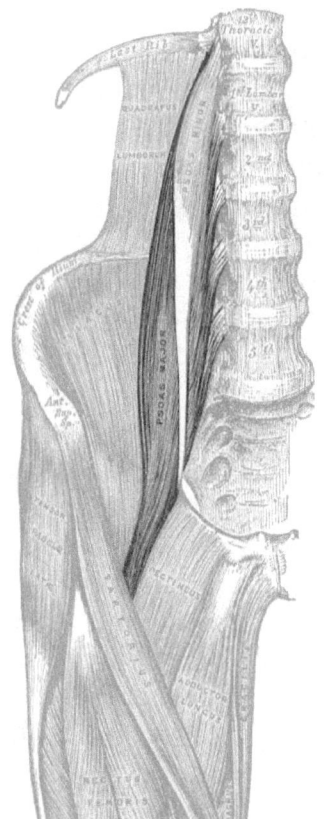

Figure 31: The psoas major, highlighted in the muscles of the groin and pelvis (Gray's Anatomy).

Let's move up to the back. As I said, the muscles in the back are just as important as those in your front. Your abs keep all that mushy stuff in your belly from falling out and they let you bend over. The psoas major lets you move your legs while you're standing or your upper body while you're lying down. But what resists that movement? How do you return from bending forward or lifting your legs up? Basically, how do you keep standing up straight (in good posture...) while you're moving around?

The main set of muscles responsible for this is called the erector spinae. This muscle set is made of three smaller sections that fan out from your spine to the middle of your back. You can feel this muscle set fairly easily if you put one hand on your spine, then feel the ropey lumps on either side of it. It helps to bend forward slightly. This is the largest of the three sections of the muscle set, and there's a matching pair, one on either side. Start from a standing posture and put your right-hand fingers on the right side of your spine and your left-hand fingers on the left side, near the small of your back. Now lean side to side, lean forward and backward, and twist your body between hips and shoulders. You should feel those ropey ridges relax and engage as you move. This band of muscle is what resists the motion of your abs in front. They don't have to be as large because they get a lot of extra support from your spine. However, if you over develop your abs and don't work on these muscles, it can lead to back problems.

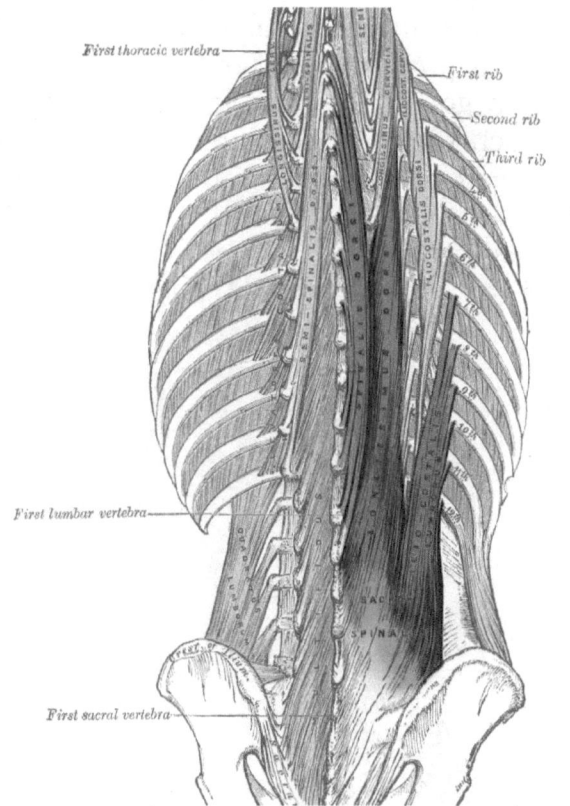

Figure 32: the erector spinae muscle group (Gray's Anatomy).

There's one other important muscle of your lower back, called the quadratus lumborum— no, that's not a spell to make a feather float. If you move your fingers out from your spine, past the erector spinae, and around your kidneys, there's another band of muscle. Technically, this is not a back muscle, but the most rearward of your abdominal muscles. It connects the top of your hip, your spine, and maybe even a rib or two (the actual connection varies from person to person). Now, you really don't want this muscle to take a lot of stress. If it is used to prop you up for long periods of time, it may get fatigued and lead to back pain. It is, in fact, the most common cause of back pain. Instead of relying on this muscle, it's better to develop your erector spinae to take the load, as that's what it's there for.

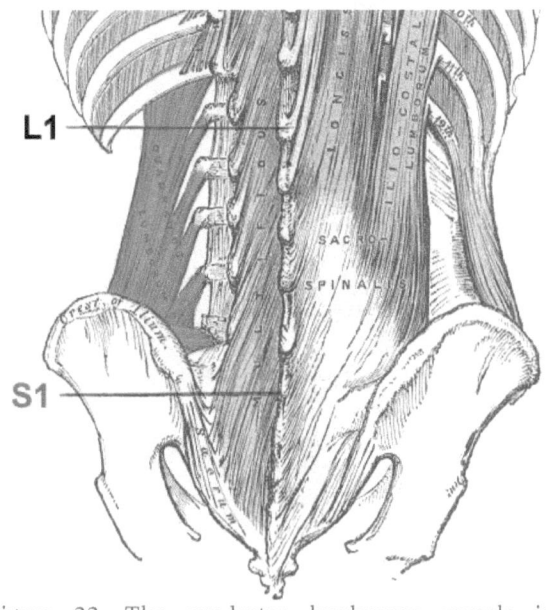

Figure 33: The quadratus lumborum muscle is highlighted (Gray's Anatomy).

Keep these abdominal muscles in mind while you move, with good posture. If you expand upward while you stand, like I've talked about, you should feel these muscles engage. Tucking your hips will keep the back muscles from compressing and losing effectiveness, and also lets your abs keep a good connection to your ribcage.

For now, I'm deliberately not going above this point on your body. There are a lot more muscles in your upper abdomen, shoulders, neck, and head, but we're going to save those for another time, because we've finally reached the main point of this book! While I have covered a few things about your arms and shoulders, the rest of this book will be concerned with your legs, leg movement, and walking. Let's dive into it.

How to walk!

We've gotten this far and I'm just now getting to how to walk? Yes. That's right. The reason it's taken so long is that I wanted you to be thinking about all the interconnected parts of your body, so you have the groundwork when I cover a complete and coordinated action, like walking. Walking does, in fact, use almost everything I've talked about so far. Even the parts you think it doesn't. *Especially* those parts.

Yes, you might think walking is easy, since you've been doing it nearly your entire life. This is false. Often while in public, I watch people walk, mostly paying attention to their feet. If you do this, you'll see there are many different methods people use to walk. Some are more efficient than others. We'll talk about that in a minute.

If you get shoulder or neck pain after walking for a long time, you probably aren't standing up straight. Go back and practice. If you are getting lower back pain, you likely aren't connected between your hips and your shoulders. Really work on tucking your hips in, and extending your upper half so you connect your hips and shoulders. Remember the exercise with your head connected by a string to the ceiling (or connected to some sort of strange skyhook if you're outside). When you don't walk as efficiently as you could, your muscles get more tired than they need to be. The section about posture at the beginning of this book is only the first step (ha). You have to practice a lot to make it innate. I've been doing

> If you've gotten to this point and you haven't done those exercises I described, **stop, go back, read them again, and try them out.** I promise that understanding—and by extension, practicing—them will make a big difference to reading the rest of this book. That is, after all, the reason you're reading it, isn't it? Otherwise, you're just nodding along with the cool things I'm saying, but not paying attention to them.

this for years and I still lose my posture.

Seriously, go back to that very first section, and practice with the timer like I said. You'll need some sense of your muscles so you understand the connection all the way from your feet to your core. Get at least a week of stretching in to start feeling some of the benefits. Relax. Set a timer along with your posture so you remember not to tense up. The worst culprits are usually shoulders and neck. Don't let your shoulders rise up into your ears.

Go on. The book will still be here when you come back.

...

Have you spent a while feeling things out? Can you recognize when you're losing your posture? Have you started stretching? If so, you may be ready to learn how to walk. Cue angelic music.

The mechanics of walking

If you've done everything above (actually done it. I've got my eye on you...), then let's go through what happens when you walk. I know you've been doing this unsupervised, with no expert in sight, for many years. Just pretend you're learning it for the first time.

Unsurprisingly, the first thing to do when trying to walk is to have good posture. You should be used to this by now and can hopefully even keep your good posture without me telling you to. But of course, I'm going to go over it again. Head up, shoulders back, hips tucked, knees slightly flexed. Pretend you have a string tying the very top of your head to the ceiling, always in tension. Extend through your core so your hips are connected to your shoulders. When you stand, reach upward, away from the ground. Think about expanding your body, rather than compacting it into a smaller space. In other words, what your mother always told you: don't hunch.

Got all that? Now we are going to walk and chew bubblegum—except I'm all out of bubblegum, so we're going to walk and hold posture.

I want you to feel the differences between efficient and inefficient movement. So, first we're going to do it the bad way. Shake everything out. Remember how you used to stand (before I came along and showered you with amazing advice).

As much as it pains me, I want you to go back to your normal posture, or even accentuate bad posture. Slump, hunch forward, have your shoulders up, head forward, hips untucked, belly out, whatever. Go for a little walk, making sure to walk forward for at least twenty feet. Try to walk backward as well and see what happens when you turn in a circle or even try to step sideways. Don't pay attention to how your feet move. We'll get to that in a minute. You might feel like you're not really getting anywhere when you walk. In fact, I hope this feels gross and awful and you never want to do it again. Because now we are going to fix it.

Even if you don't feel anything, don't worry. The next exercise should make the difference clearer.

No pressure. Stand in good posture. Head, shoulders, hips, knees, connection, extension.

I want you to go for a little walk. Don't pay attention to your feet yet. Just worry about keeping that posture and connection intact. Don't even take this book with you because I don't want you to be looking down (but read the rest of this paragraph and the next first so you know what you're doing). Look straight forward when you walk so you don't tilt your head up or down and accidentally ruin your posture.

Here's what I want you to do: walk about twenty feet forward, then stop and walk backward. One of the things I always find hardest is keeping your hips tucked while you're walking. Make sure they don't sag and lose connection with your core and shoulders. Next, turn in a complete circle with your head still upright in good posture (remember that posture). Finally try stepping sideways. Go do this, then come back and read the next section.

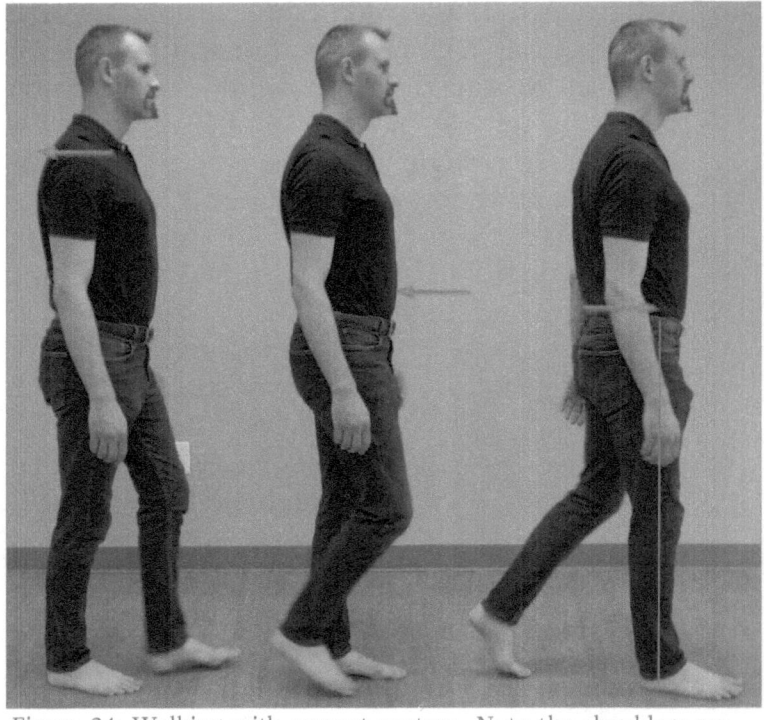

Figure 34: Walking with correct posture. Note the shoulders are back, the abs are connected to the hips and shoulders, and the center moves forward while walking, and is above the newly planted foot.

How did you do? Did it feel different than the first time? If you've gone from having no connection to full connection, walking should feel a lot "lighter," more fluid, and more coordinated than what you did before. You may feel like you're walking slower, yet covering the same distance you used to. Why? Because you've aligned your center of balance underneath you, rather than in front of you. You've also created a light connection all the way from your feet to your shoulders. You're not fully tense, but you're not completely relaxed either. Especially when moving backward, sideways, or turning, you should feel it's much easier to adjust your direction because your center of mass is closer to where all the action is happening: your hips.

Remember how I said everything is about your hips? Does that make more sense now? While getting your upper body posture correct is challenging, I find being aware of how your hips move is even harder and takes a lot longer to master.

Let's go back to the description of finding the center of mass for a minute. You don't need to actually hang yourself up on a wall, but if you imagine yourself in a flat plane (standing straight, with good posture) rather than in a curve (slumped forward), you can visualize that the center of your mass will be on the flat plane you make by standing up, rather than out in space in the middle of the curve from your hips to your head. Notice the straight line in Figure 35. It starts in the same place on the foot, but goes through the middle of the hip and the middle of the ear on the picture with good posture, and through neither on the one with poor posture.

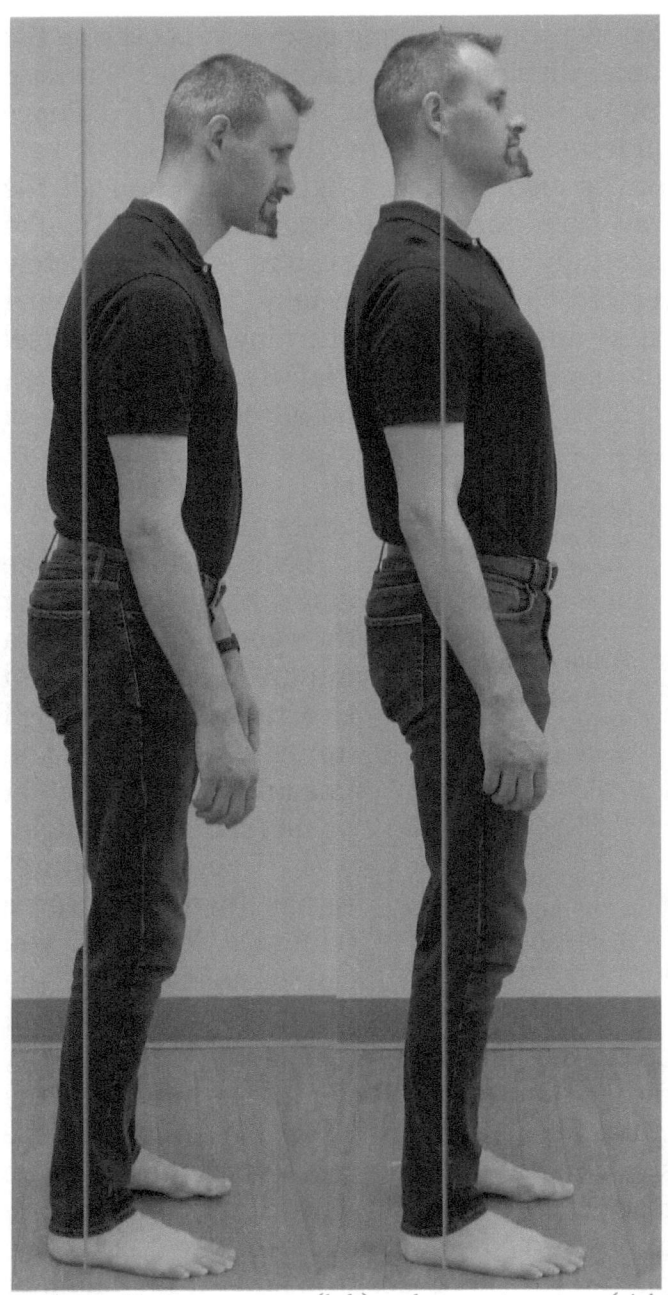

Figure 35: Poor posture (left) and correct posture (right). Notice the center of mass (red line) goes through the heel, waist, and ear when in correct posture.

On the other hand, if visualizing stuff like this makes your head hurt, don't worry about it. Just remember, if your body is in a straight line rather than a curve, then it's easier to move.

We're going to get into more complex analysis from here on out, and I want to make sure you have the fundamentals down— the fundamentals being everything up to this point. And you thought walking was easy.

Time to practice again. I don't mind if you put the book down at this point and simply work on absorbing this concept for a week or so. You can just...uh...walk away from it.

Try to combine walking with the timer you use for posture and relaxation. You want to do all three at the same time (you can do all three at once, right?) so you don't put any extra effort into walking. Efficiency comes from the least energy input for the maximum work output. You can walk longer, farther, or with less stress on your body by using less energy to do it.

Try to walk and hold posture. You're still all out of bubblegum. Go practice again and try to remember all the things I've talked about. Good posture, hip to shoulder connection, relaxation, keeping your center in line, least effort. Try to keep all of this in mind. Okay, go on and take a walk.

I'll wait here.

...

Don't worry, I'm still waiting.

...

Have you practiced your walking? If you've done this over a period of several days, then are you starting to make this a habit? Does your walking gait feel better? Can you go faster with little effort? You might find yourself passing people who are suddenly walking so slowly. If you *have* practiced, everything I've talked about should start to become second nature. I hope it has, because we're really going into the deep end now. Deep breath.

How your feet move when walking

I told you to ignore your feet in the last part for a reason. I have a whole section about it here, so let's talk about your feet. Now you're aware of the basics (lots of them!) of walking, were going to break down some tangential parts and see how they affect the whole.

This part will be easier to do without shoes, but if you have them on, that's fine. Just make sure you pay attention to what the different parts of your feet are doing in your shoes. Whenever you get a chance, try the same exercises with bare feet.

How do your feet contact the ground when you walk? Do you go heel-toe, heel-toe?

Humans have walked in different manners throughout history, but for right now, in a society where we use shoes that have good support and are long-lasting, I'm going to say that heel-toe is the best method for how your feet should contact the ground during a regular walking gait. Let's look at some of the other methods in comparison. A lot of the inefficiencies I see in people walking come from putting your feet to the floor in a different sequence.

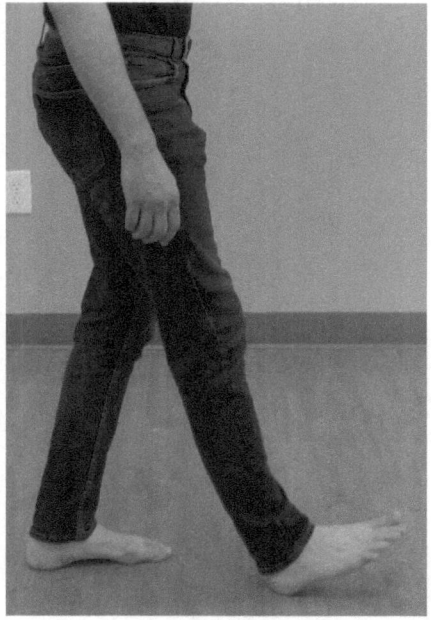

Figure 36: Walking heel-toe.

Some put their full foot on the floor at one time, stomping around with every step. It's more common with people who are hunched forward. If you use good posture, this is actually pretty hard to do because placing the full length of your foot on the ground at one time means your center of mass needs to be over the center of your foot. If you have good posture, your center of mass is going to be nearer your heel. Walking with the full flat of your foot also reduces the amount of flex through your foot, which can be bad for your tendons and for your knees. Wearing shoes that don't bend or are worn out might make this issue worse. If you're not able to roll your foot from heel to toe when touching the floor because it's encased in a heavy, unyielding material, you're more likely to walk flat-footed.

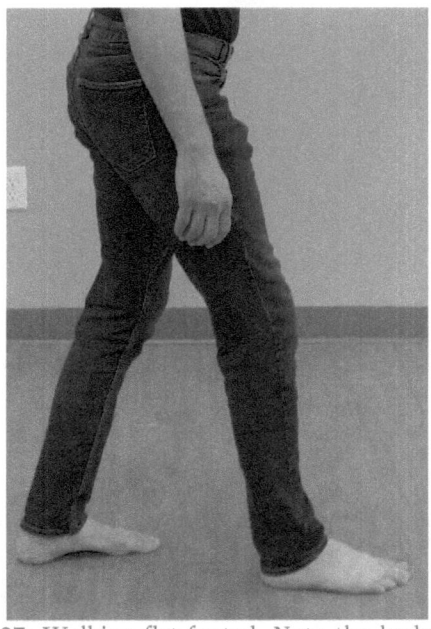

Figure 37: Walking flat-footed. Note the body above the waist is bent forward more.

Others walk on their toes, which, while good for some types of running (and for being sneaky), is not as beneficial for walking. When walking like this, your Achilles tendon (remember, that's the big springy thing that connects your heel to your leg) gets very tight. You can even strain it by walking on your toes for long periods of time. On the other hand (foot?), walking on your toes for short periods of time can work on your balance and muscle tension. But just like lifting weights, you don't want to do it all the time. If you've walked in high heels for hours or even minutes, you probably understand this.

If you walk in heels, the Achilles tendon is shortened and relaxed, passively. Standing on tiptoes is done by contracting the tendon, so it's active. Thus, an Achilles tendon strain can be treated using cowboy boots, which shorten and relax the tendon.

Another point worth mentioning is that walking toe-heel, or even only on the toes, is common among neurodivergent people. As I've said above, there's good reason to work on changing this walking method if you do it. Aside from issues with the Achilles tendon tightening, you can see in the comparison below how it affects your balance and efficiency (see Figure 38).

The method of walking that's hardest to diagnose, and the one I find most insidious in terms of ruining your posture and walking gait, is "bouncing" while you walk. This method is hard to see. If you look at someone's feet while they walk, your eye naturally goes to the foot that's taking a step, rather than the one that's still on the ground. Your eyes are attracted to movement. If you force yourself to focus on the foot that stays on the floor, you may see the heel pop up before the person finishes the next step. This little "pop" while walking causes all manner of inefficiencies and breaks your connection with the ground, and with your posture.

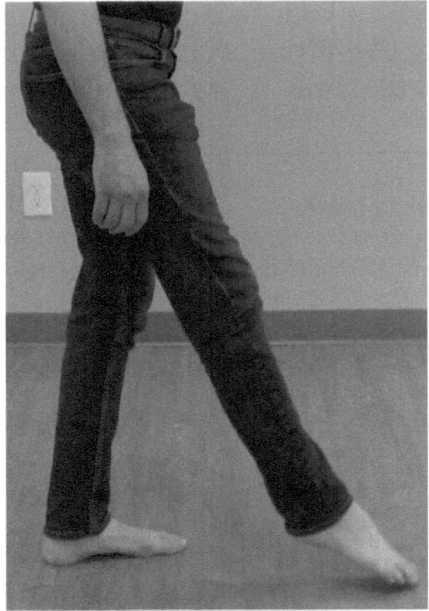

Figure 38: Walking toe-heel. Note the center is more over the back foot.

Remember how I said efficiency means using the least energy to do the most work? If you pop or bounce while you walk, you're doing more work in order to get the same job done. That "pop" in your stationary foot means even if you have good posture, you're rocking your whole body forward over the front of your foot. Can you imagine where your center of mass goes as you do this? To maintain posture, if you're even able to, you would have to pull your entire weight back from your toes to your heel.

While it's a shift of maybe six or seven inches, you're shifting your entire mass backward while your intention is to walk forward. You're putting energy into going in the opposite direction to the one you want to. Most people who walk this way don't even try to correct their posture, as most of them aren't aware they're doing this.

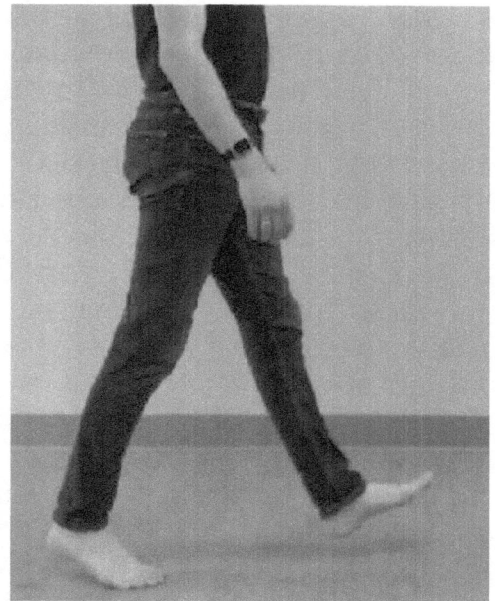

Figure 39: Walking with a bounce or "pop." Note the center is disconnected from the ground.

Instead, the person leans forward while walking and is forced to use their back muscles to compensate for their head being over their toes rather than over their heels. If they already have a slump forward in their neck and shoulders, this only exacerbates the problem. I guess what I'm saying, in short, is: don't walk this way.

Now that I've gone through (or ranted about) some of the ways you shouldn't walk, let's try heel to toe walking. This is going to feel silly, like something you already know how to do, but stay with me. Even if you don't think you need to do this, try it out, just in case.

Start, as always, with good posture. Remember to tuck those hips. Now, *without moving your upper body, or leaning or moving forward at all*, put one foot out in front of you, heel pointing down to the floor and toes raised at about a 30-degree angle from the floor. Let your heel settle to the floor. You'll probably have to shift your balance sideways over your support leg just a little to keep from leaning. Also, since you haven't moved your center of mass forward, you may also feel tension in your rear leg. That's because we've only done half of what you need to do to take a step.

Let's add the second part. Go back to where you were, standing up straight with your feet together. Now when you put the foot out in front of you, move your hips over your rear foot until they are over your toes instead of your heel. This will look a lot like Figure 36. You are shifting your balance forward while you do this, as well as shifting sideways to balance as you did

> Tldr:
> Step 1: put your foot out without shifting your hips forward.
> Step 2: Do the same thing, but shift your hips forward this time. You'll feel your weight settle differently.

in the first example. In order to keep your balance and keep from falling, your heel will land on the ground. Do you feel the difference between moving your center and not moving your center?

This is why I talked about your hips and your center of balance so much at the beginning of the book. They are central (quite literally) to how you walk.

Let's take a different example, just to show you why I like heel-toe better than the other methods of foot movement. Do what you did the first time—stand up straight and reach one foot out, but this time instead of pointing your heel at the floor, point your toes at the floor. When you touch the floor with your toes, you'll notice there isn't as much pressure on the rear leg as there is when you touch with your heel. You also don't really have to move your center. This is why it's good for sneaking around (see the explanation in the box). You don't have to commit your center to the movement, and you can test the ground where you're going to take a step.

But for these purposes, if you walk toe-heel, toe-heel instead of the other way around, you put less pressure on the back leg and you don't move your center forward. You *can* move your

> Watch how far you put your foot out when taking a step. You don't need to take a giant step, but your stride should be just long enough so you do have to move your center forward while stepping. If you don't move your center, you can step very quietly, but won't get anywhere fast.

120   William C. Tracy

center forward if you walk this way, though you're less likely to, naturally. So why do I not prefer this method of walking? Because you *want* some tension between your body parts. Think of the stretching exercises, especially the isometrics. Creating a little tension can show you the most efficient line of motion. The muscles that get tense indicate you're at the extent of your available movement and must now move other parts of your body to continue.

When you have pressure that makes you move your hips forward, you will innately start to shift them forward earlier in the step. Why is this necessary? Because when you move parts of your body in coordination, rather than one after the other, it's more efficient.

Let's try one more example to show you why I prefer heel-toe. I'm going to make you imitate the dreaded heel popping. Oh no! Those who walk this way, I'm glaring at you (you can't see it, but I am).

> The total energy to move two body parts together is less than moving them one at a time. This is a more difficult concept to grasp, so if you don't fully get it, don't worry yet. We're still just focusing on your feet.

By now, you should know to start with good posture. Like we did in the first example, stick one foot out, heel pointing toward the floor, move your hips in, and let your heel land. So far, so good. Here's that insidious balance shift that comes along with popping. I want you to *keep* shifting your balance over your front foot and lift up your rear heel up at the same time. You're standing on the toes of your rear foot and the heel of your front foot, and as you roll to put your front foot flat on the ground, your center must shift farther than normal and end up over your front toes. See Figure 39 for reference. So even before you finish your step, your center is too far forward. When you bring your back leg through, your center of mass is over the toes of your stationary foot rather than over the heel. It's as if you're continuously falling forward. The only way to stop this is to bring your entire body backward as I described above, which takes more energy than necessary.

To make this even worse, most people don't have good posture (like you do, after all that practice!). So, try the same example as above, but this time, lean your shoulders and head forward (like I told you not to) as you step. If you pop your rear heel up as you are walking, and your shoulders and

> Aside from inefficiency, there's one other reason I despise "pop" walking. One key word: fall. You should always be in control of where your body is moving, but while walking with a "pop" you're falling forward because you're not in control of your center.

head are forward, your balance will be even farther forward, and you cannot help but fall onto your new foot, often sending a shock through your front leg. This is bad on your Achilles tendon and your knees, as well as being inefficient. This method of walking encourages you to have bad posture in order to fall into your next step. You are never completely in control of your motion.

Hopefully these examples explain why I like walking heel-toe. If not, read through the section above again. Go very slowly and feel out what I'm describing. Look at the pictures and compare them to what you're doing. There are a lot of subtle complexities, and it may well take a few read-throughs and trying it out for yourself to understand.

Now, try the heel-to-toe method. Good posture, from head to shoulders to hips and knees. Feel where your center of mass is, and as you take a step, move your center of mass *with* your front foot moving rather than before

Time for a pop quiz! I did say there would be a test later. Which way do you walk? If you don't naturally walk heel-toe, try to figure out why. Are you not moving your hips forward when you walk? Are you leaning forward? Are you popping and falling forward? Feel how your thighs, glutes, and core move. Take twenty or thirty minutes to go over these different walking methods and try to understand how they do and do not work. You may have corrected some of your worst habits already if you've been practicing with correct posture. At least that's my hope.

or after it moves. As soon as you pick up your front foot, your hips should also start forward.

Congratulations! You just took your first step (ha ha!) toward walking efficiently!

Using both legs to walk

Before moving on to this section, take some time to process the sections above. There's a lot crammed in there. Even if you set this book down for a week or two and try everything out, that's fine. Especially if you're making changes to your stance and the way you walk at the same time—for example getting rid of the habit of popping while you walk—it can take a while before your body gets used to it. Don't worry. The book will still be here.

Remember what I said at the very beginning: from posture, to body connection from your feet to your head, to the way you place your feet when you walk, I've covered some major adjustments to how you operate your body. Once all those changes start to gel, *then* it's time to move on to the rest of this book. From here on, we are going to refine ever smaller pieces of how you move to get the maximum efficiency.

What helps the most in learning to do something new or different with your body is to *feel* what your body is doing as you move. You won't understand how to truly operate your collection of bones, muscles, and organs unless you know exactly what each muscle is doing. You don't have to know the fancy names or anything, as long as you pay attention to how you move. As I practice martial arts and body kinematics, even when I'm just walking around, I sometimes go down to the level of tensing and contracting one muscle at a time to figure out what it does and how it affects my body. You don't need to do this, because you're reading this book and I'm sharing some of the things I've learned. But if do you want to try this out, it's a good way to get in tune with your body.

...

Did you take some time to learn the above techniques?

You've have had a lot of new concepts thrown at you. If you're used to hunching over a computer at work, learn to sit up straight and use your core when you get up and sit down. If you stand at your job a lot, see if you can be more efficient when you walk from place to place. Try to keep your feet from getting tired by working on different muscles.

Go for a walk and practice out these techniques! Walk heel-toe, toe-heel, and pop. No one is watching you. No one at all.

Here's a benchmark to see if you've got the basics:

1) Can you feel where your center is at all times?
2) Can you feel good posture and bad posture?
3) Can you keep good posture while moving?
4) Do you know which method you'd been using to walk (before you started practicing heel-toe)?

...

At the very least, take two or three days and
practice your posture and stepping heel to
toe while moving your center. I'll wait.

These can be techniques you use the rest of
your life! Taking a few days to learn them is
worth it.

If you're sure you're ready to move on, here's
one more check: can you successfully take a
few steps heel-toe, in good posture, *while*
moving your center with your motion?

If so, read on.

...

Ok. Now it's time to dive into something more subtle. Let's move on to using *both* legs while you walk. I bet you thought you were doing this already, but you probably weren't. At least not as well as you could. For example, do you walk slow or fast? If most people pass you as you walk, you can increase your speed by using both legs instead of just one to help yourself along. I'll explain what this means.

Let's do the example from the previous section. Stand straight, get a good connection in your center, one foot out in front, heel down, move your center forward, plant your foot, repeat. Got it? Good.

Let's add some more muscles into this. I want you to take a step as above and pause when your front foot hits the floor *while* your rear foot is still fully planted (with even the heel touching—no popping!). You should feel tension between your legs, or maybe a stretch in your back calf. From here, pull into the center of your body with the rear of your front thigh (your hamstring on the stepping foot) and the front of your rear thigh (your quadriceps on the foot that will step next). You'll feel the pressure increase between your legs. Keep shifting your balance (your center) over your front foot and lift your back foot very slightly off the floor. It starts to swing forward on its own, doesn't it? That's good.

Try this again. Take one heel-toe step, plant both feet, squeeze your thighs together, release your back foot, and *as your back foot moves forward,* use this extra momentum to swing your new leg forward to plant it heel-toe in your next step.

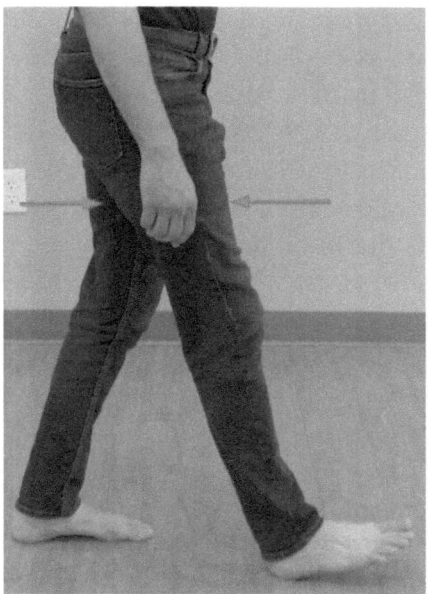

Figure 40: Use the muscles in both legs to walk, squeezing in along the red arrows before releasing your back foot from the floor.

Here's another important concept: as your rear foot swings forward, *now* is the time to release the tension in your thighs. If you keep this tension up it will restrict your movement rather than helping it, so it's important to relax in the middle of taking a step.

Tensing then relaxing afterward is a hard concept to practice and you probably won't get it right away. That's fine. Just keep it in mind as you continue working on using both legs to walk.

Take a few minutes to practice and see if you can adapt the

movement from jerky, stuttering steps to more fluid motion. Practice tensing, then relaxing your legs. If you need to, take out the walking part of this and pause in the middle of a step, with one leg in front of the other. Practice tensing your front hamstring and rear quad, then release. Do it ten or twenty times until you get the idea, even if it's not perfect. Once you've got that, come back here and read on.

No really, go practice. You should be used to this by now.

Oh, and fix your posture. Yeah, I know.

...

Okay, ready to move on?

Now that you have the idea of this "step-squeeze-release-relax" motion, let's add yet *one more* layer of complexity (there's always one more...).

In the middle of your step, after you squeeze your thighs, as you release your rear foot from the floor, *keep* moving your hips (and thus your center) forward to the toes of your front foot. Your rear leg will move even farther forward. I know it sounds like I've already said this, but I promise it's different. The difference is subtle. You can check by looking straight down after the step. Your bellybutton should be directly between your feet, rather than at the toes of (what is now) your rear foot. If this sounds confusing, just try to walk and make sure you keep your center moving as you do it.

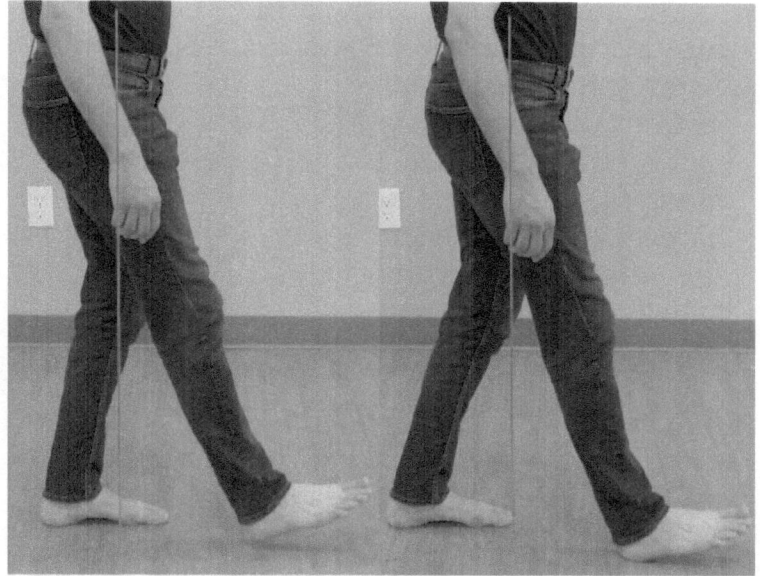

Figure 41: Left: stepping with the center of mass over the center of the back foot. Right: stepping with the center of mass over the toe of the back foot.

Go practice again, then come back so I can add one more detail (I told you there was always one more).

...

Okay, last time, really (for this section). Good posture, step forward heel-toe, squeeze your thighs, release, relax, move your center forward. Got all that? It's a lot to keep in your brain at once. Once you start to break this down to individual muscles, even very simple movements can turn out to be very complex. Your brain has learned over time how to do them without you thinking about them, and now you're breaking that pattern.

The final part is to keep moving your center forward even *past* your support foot as you swing your new leg out in front. Because if you move your center forward, you're going to have to compensate for the new placement by taking a larger step. This is the same thing you do when you start running, but we're doing it while you're walking. This means your walking stride is going to get longer, and you are going to take bigger steps. Thus, you will be able to walk faster. We're taking the mechanism of running and turning it into controlled walking!

> It can be frustrating to break things down like this, but I promise it will feel really good when you finally put it back together.

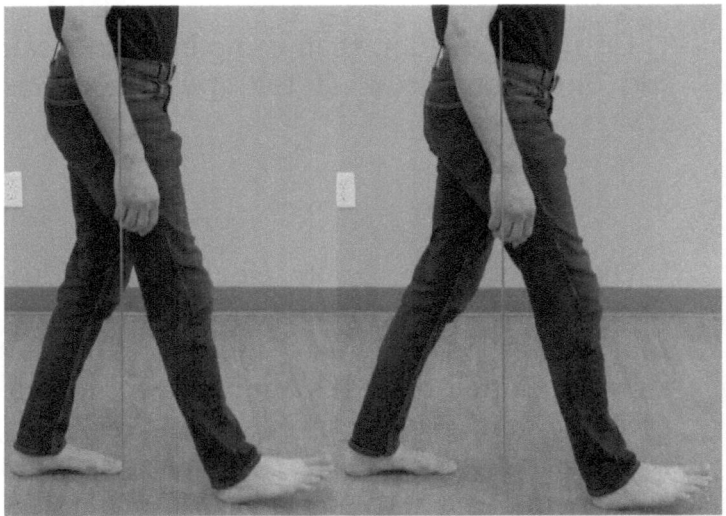

Figure 42: Left: stepping with the center of mass over the toe of the back foot. Right: Stepping with the center of mass past the toe of the back foot.

Throughout all this, remember your posture! You're likely looking down at your feet as you walk. Where's that bowling ball? Once you know where your center is going, pull your shoulders back and head up as you walk. Look directly forward, and you should have better control and balance.

All this may feel very mechanical as you practice, especially if you're feeling things out. That's fine to start. Try the motion, even if it feels clunky and robotic. Do each step as I've outlined, without blending them together yet. That comes later, after you're sure your muscles are operating in the correct manner and you've retrained your brain, just like any other sort of practice.

Slowly speed your walk up as you get more comfortable with this long stride. Eventually, you'll be taking full, heel-toe steps and using both of your legs to propel your motion. Are you remembering your posture as you go faster? It's easy to bring your shoulders and head forward because that makes it seem like you're covering more ground. But resist that feeling. If you keep your head and shoulders above your center while you move, I promise you will actually be able to move faster. Even better, you will be able to stop, reverse, and change directions much quicker. This is helpful for not running into walls, or people, or tripping over pets with your new super speed.

Just like everything else, all this will take time to learn. It's all right to put this book down for a while and let your body process the changes you're making. There's a thing called muscle memory, which comes from doing an action so many times it's ingrained in the part of your brain that deals with reflexes rather than voluntary action. Athletes, musicians, or really anyone who does a repetitive task will find those processes moved to muscle memory. It's the same thing as learning to touch type. When your fingers know where the keys are, you don't have to think about which one you're pressing.

There is a *lot* to unpack in this chapter—more than in the rest of the book combined. It's okay to feel overwhelmed. It's okay to go back to a section and say, "I really didn't understand that part." Look at the pictures included with this book. They are another form of input and may make more sense than trying to digest a lot of words strung together.

Here are some tips and tricks to consider as you adapt your walking gait:

- The more you move your center forward while you take a step, the faster you will go. Eventually, you will turn the motion into running. Check this by running, then walking, to see the difference.

- Practice your posture and remember to keep up a connection while you walk. It's incredibly easy to forget. I do so on a regular basis, and I've been doing this for years. Always remember your hips, keeping them tucked, and keeping a connection to your core muscles. To check, you shouldn't be able to completely relax your abs while standing.

- See how fast you can walk while maintaining your motion and posture. Depending on your leg length, you may be able to take much bigger steps than you're used to. You also may hit the limit of how far your legs can comfortably reach. Always check that you can stop quickly and safely (within 1-2 steps) from a full walk!
- Make sure you don't overbalance and start to fall. You're learning to walk a second time, and you haven't done this since you were a toddler. Mistakes will happen! Check that your head is always above your center of mass.

Changing something so fundamental to how you move takes a lot of time to reprocess and relearn, and I've thrown a lot of information at you in this section. I know how hard it is, as I've had to relearn ingrained techniques several times while training in martial arts. It's never an easy process and can even take *years* to do. The key is dedication, and remembering to go slowly while you learn. *Only* speed things up when you're sure you have the motion down. To test yourself, speed up to the point where something "breaks," that is, your posture goes, or you stumble, or something else. When you reach this point, you know you've gone too far, and need to bring your speed down in order to get better at that motion. Practice some more, then speed things up again and see if you can go a little bit faster before things break. Pretty soon you'll be speed walking with the best of them!

Side issues in walking

Slumping

Yes, I've covered this a lot, but I want to reiterate the importance of posture, now you've read the most challenging parts. One of the most insidious and difficult-to-combat posture issues is slumping. I use this as a catchall term for the type of posture where you're sitting down, your neck is forward, and your stomach is hanging out. I'm not talking about whether you have a belly or flat abs, but whether your core is engaged, even if you're sitting down. Especially with the prevalence of office jobs, a lot of people nowadays sit for the better part of the day. When sitting for long periods of time, you want to relax, and that leads to letting the chair support you rather than sitting *up* in the chair.

But even when you relax, don't slump so the wrong muscles have to take up the slack. If you're standing up and tilting forward, your back structure has to compensate for lost posture, especially if you let your hips tip forward. The same thing applies in a

To clarify, I'm not saying you can never relax. You certainly can. Lean back in a chair, watch some TV, play a video game, listen to some music. Or when you're standing, lean against a wall and take a load off. But when you're actively engaged in an activity, try to keep your core engaged and your posture good.

chair, because if you slump, you are letting your hips disengage the connection in your abdomen. In this case, because your hips can't move anywhere, it's felt by your belly going soft and no longer holding your shoulders up. At this point, you start leaning forward, your neck juts out, and your shoulders roll forward. If you add to that holding a cell phone in your hand, it's very easy to lean your head forward so that you're looking down into your lap, thus exacerbating the problem.

The way to combat this is to always be aware of the posture I've discussed (ad nauseam) in this book. If you practice to the point where you know you have a connection all the way from your shoulders to your toes, you can keep that connection whether you're standing, sitting, or lying down. Okay, I'll relent on that last one. You can relax when you're asleep.

As with everything else, be aware of what you're doing. If you start to encapsulate the lessons of this book, you may suddenly find you are aware when you're slumping. If you know you're doing something not good for your body, it's a lot easier to address the issue. That leads to the next topic.

Sitting Up and Sitting Down

As identified above, good posture is not limited to when standing up. It's also very important while you're sitting down. The posture and connection I've been talking about have to become second nature, so much so that you maintain them in transitions as well, and not just while you are stationary.

Let's talk about one of the most common transitions, which is sitting down and standing back up. When you sit down, try not to flop into the chair you're sitting in. Instead, practice keeping the connection all the way down to the seat. It's going to feel a lot different, and it's going to take a little bit more musculature in your thighs.

Try it out now. I'll wait here.

How did sitting down feel? It always makes me feel very regal, as if I'm holding court while trying to sit down. This is, of course, because you're now doing it with correct posture and acting all refined.

> "Flopping" is a function of suddenly letting go of the connection between your hips and your shoulders, anticipating that the chair will take the load. If you simply don't have enough muscle to support yourself, try this: put both hands on your thighs and slide them to your knees as you sit down, pressing into your legs. This can make a connection that helps you keep your core engaged.

So, what about the other direction, when you want to stand back up? Do you bend forward so your shoulders come over the edge of the chair and sort of fall out of it until you can stand up? This is what most people do, but now you know about your center of mass, you know what's happening. When you lean your shoulders forward, you're moving your center of mass enough so it's now over your feet or your toes.

Then it only takes a little bit of effort to stand up. This is all well and good, but don't make this a substitute for using the connection between your hips and your shoulders to help you stand.

Instead of rolling forward, keep that good posture and connection, and tilt your whole upper body forward. You still get the desired effect of changing your center of mass so it's over your feet and you can stand up. You'll also, again, use a little bit more muscle in your thighs to stand up.

Try these two methods out:

First, from a seated position, roll forward without good posture until you can "fall upward."

Next, keep your posture and lean forward before standing. If you need to, you can press your hands into your thighs to help push yourself up. If you have good posture, you may find it takes a much smaller shift to bring your shoulders forward to where you can stand up easily. And you thought walking was hard!

Walking on the sides of your feet

Let's talk about less common aspects of people's walking gaits. The first is rolling your feet to the outside or inside while you walk. I don't have hard evidence to back this up, but I suspect if your feet rest more naturally at an open angle, you're more inclined to walk on the insides of your feet. On the other hand, if your toes tend to point toward each other at rest, you may be prone to walking on the outsides of your feet. Walking on the insides of your feet, to me, is the more ergonomically worrying position. When you do this, your knees have a tendency to buckle inward, which can cause strain on the tendons and ligaments in that area. There is also little musculature support on the inside of your foot where the arch is.

Walking on the outside of your foot is also something to be avoided, if possible. This puts strain on the outside of the knee rather than inside, although you have more support because you can still use your toes to grip the floor. There are some martial arts stances that actually have you stand on the "ridge edge" of your feet. Walking this way all the time, however, means you must divert extra effort to keeping your balance.

> Remember I said way back in the anatomy section that I would be talking later about moving on the sides of your feet? This still isn't it!

Wobbling

There are several different ways people wobble to the sides when they walk rather than moving forward in a straight line. Often, it's when people are taking their ease, and simply not walking very fast, enjoying the view. The tendency here is to shift your body over one foot and then over the other, as this diverts momentum from going forward and makes you slow down. I'm not as concerned about this one, as it does sort of make sense. You don't have any particular place to be, and you aren't concerned about being incredibly efficient while you walk. That's fine.

There are some other forms of wobbling that seem to be more of a habit for people. Moving your shoulders side to side, or one shoulder forward then the other, while you walk seems intimidating. You are swaggering or showing off that you're in control. But to do this all the time when you're trying to get somewhere is counterintuitive. You waste a lot of energy doing so and you are less stable on your feet. If you *were* trying to intimidate someone, you're actually *more* susceptible to being pushed over!

Finally, if you keep your weight too far backward while you walk (so that your center is more than that two fingers behind your bellybutton), then you're going to fall into a sort of swaying rhythm, where your hips move over one foot then the other while you walk. Again, this keeps you from moving forward as efficiently as you could.

There may be reasons to wobble while walking. Just be aware that every time you shift your body to the side rather than shifting forward, you're decreasing your walking efficiency.

Head bobbing

This last issue is concerned with connection, but not between your hips and your shoulders. It's the connection between your shoulders and your head. You may see people do this, or may even have done it yourself, where you walk almost like a pigeon, bobbing your head forward with every step. If you follow the good posture like I covered throughout this book, your ears are going to be over your shoulders. If this is the case, then you shouldn't be able to bob your head forward. If you let your head fall forward or are looking at a cell phone in your hand for example, your head may start to bob simply from the up-and-down motion of walking. It's fairly easy to correct this if you reset to a good posture: ears over your shoulders, shoulders back, hips tucked, knees slightly bent, feet straight in front of you.

You are not a velociraptor. Don't head bob while you're walking, as if looking for prey (or a cell signal). Hold your cellphone up higher if needed.

I am certain there are many more side issues I could get into, but this is all I'm going to cover for now. Mainly because I want to get to the last section in this book, which is one of my favorites. If you've practiced everything to this point, you'll have a good handle on keeping your posture steady, keeping your core engaged, and moving your center forward while you walk. Let's use those principles to get into the fun things you can do while learning how to operate your body.

Body Mechanics Tips and Tricks

In this last section, I'm going to go over a few cool tips and tricks that don't fit elsewhere. These aren't in any particular order, but you may find them useful in certain situations. Some use your arms, some use your legs. If nothing else, just let them percolate through your brain and see if any of them stick since you're now a master of walking efficiently!

Fast and loose vs. slow and steady movement

The temptation when you're able to move more efficiently, is to also move faster. This is not always the best plan, as the faster you move, the more you lose the posture and connection you've been trying to develop.

When you're learning a new skill, remember to start out slow. Even if you feel silly, or aren't progressing as fast as somebody else, remember there's no reason to compare yourself against others. If you can do a skill just as well

If you've ever practiced a musical instrument or other physical activity, you're probably aware of how making slow movements and speeding up can lead to better results than trying to learn at a faster speed.

slowly as you can fast, then you're well on your way to mastering it.

I always tell my martial arts students I would rather see a form performed slowly and correctly rather than fast and sloppily. When you move slowly, you are also able to weed out inbuilt inefficiencies that are hard to see when you move fast. The total learning time may end up being *shorter* than if you go fast and mess things up. Just keep in mind as you move about life that *fast is not always the best option*. Better if you start out slow, and work on a skill until you're able to do it either slow or fast.

Muscles moving against each other

Your muscles don't move in isolation. Since you suspend yourself vertically and against gravity while standing, you naturally use some muscles more than others, especially when you stand up. As Newton said, for every action there is an equal and opposite reaction. This means when you push against something, that something will push

I covered this concept briefly in the sections on connection and isometrics, but I wanted to expand on the topic now that you've gone through the rest of the exercises. I'm going to give you some examples about using muscular tension to offset everyday back against you. This is also true inside your body.

When you push with one arm, there's going to be a reaction, and if you don't balance yourself, you'll turn in a circle. You already know how to compensate, but we can take this concept and turn it into an advantage rather than simply resisting gravity.

Try this: stand in front of an open doorway, and push with one hand into one side of the doorframe. You can feel the stress all the way down your legs into the ground, because you're compensating for not rotating away from the doorframe where you pushed it. Now put one hand on either side of the doorframe and push equally. You only need to resist the backward motion. Obvious, right? Let's try a more complicated example.

Go back to that same doorway, and this time hook just your fingers around the doorframe so you can pull yourself to one side. If you only pull with one hand, then you have to resist being pulled over. Now let's do the same second part as before. Wrap fingers of one hand around either side of the doorframe. If you pull equally with both hands, you stay where you are, and as a bonus, the rest of your body doesn't have to resist falling over. Muscles are moving against each other to keep you in place. You can put as much force as you want to into one hand, and still resist that force with the other hand. Newton is proven correct once again.

I know these seem like silly examples, but I want you to understand the idea because this is a sort of nebulous concept. Let's try something more complex. Say you're trying to hammer a nail into a wall. If you stand completely still and try to move the hammer only with your forearm, you're only going to get so much force out of it. Feel free to try this, but please find a safe and inconspicuous surface first. Don't blame this book for holes in your walls.

Once you've got the idea, try hammering again, but this time let your upper body move with the motion so that your off shoulder (the one you're not using to hammer with) starts moving as well. Because you are now moving both sides of your body, you can coordinate the timing so that you get much more force in each hammering motion. It's sort of a whip-like action, passing through your upper body.

How about a less...destructive example? Say you're getting food out of the fridge and setting it on the counter. You either open the fridge with your dominant hand and pick up the item with your non-dominant hand, or vice versa. Now you have two things you need to do: you need to put the food down somewhere, and you also need to close the fridge.

Rather than make this two separate actions, make it the same action. Use the action that requires more force—closing the fridge—as a counterbalance to get your body moving in the right direction to put the food down on the counter. Rather than waste energy moving one direction, then moving in another direction, use Newton's action and reaction to reposition yourself where you need to be. When you push the door closed, let that force aid you in moving away from it toward your destination.

However, in order to do so, you must have a good connection through your body and core. That way, you're not wasting energy by twisting your body, when you could be using that energy to swing a foot in the direction you want to go. I could go on this topic for a long time, as it ties in strongly with what I teach in my martial arts class. For now, try redirecting energy into the next action that you do.

> I guess you technically don't have to have good posture for this, but I hope you do after reading the rest of this book.

Completing a circle

Let's move on to the concept of completing a circle with your body. It's related to moving your muscles against each other. If you can create a circle with your limbs, you're able to use more of the maximum strength of your body.

Here's an easy example. Try to lift a

> I'm not going to go deep into the mechanical reasons behind this, but I believe it has to do with your kinesthetic sense. That is, knowing where your limbs are. If you have two limbs occupied in the same action, the dual feedback to your brain helps it interpret the data more accurately.

heavy object with one arm. Now add the other arm to it, even without adding its full strength. You may suddenly be able to lift the object. It's the same idea as if you try to steady a hand that's doing a precise action, by touching it with your other hand.

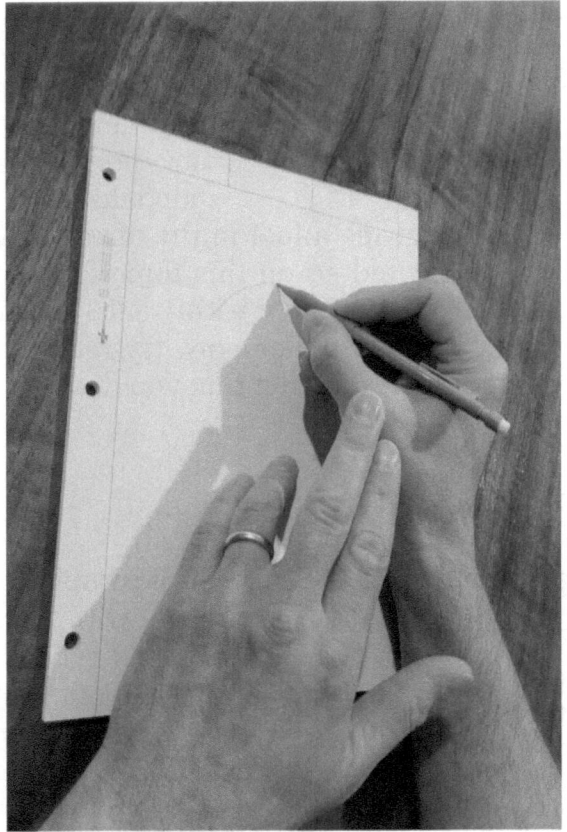

Figure 43: Touching one side of your body to the other can give greater fine control of action.

On the physical side, if you use both halves of your body in an action, it becomes easier to balance, or to offset the weight of the object you're dealing with.

The combination of this physical and mental feedback means you're better able to compensate for any errors while you do whatever it is you're doing.

Here's another example. Try standing on one foot. At first, keep the foot in the air from touching anything else. Depending on your balance, standing on one foot may be hard or easy. Now try touching the foot in the air to the grounded leg. You may notice your balance suddenly gets better, or you can hold the pose for longer. You now have the feedback from both of your legs rather than just one. Try this out in different situations and see if you can feel your body reacting to the feedback of two limbs rather than one.

A harder example than above, mainly because not a lot of people can do them, is pull-ups. If you can do one, try doing a pull-up with your feet separate, then a pull-up with your feet touching. You may find the second way is easier.

It's a fairly simple idea that it is easier to do something if your muscles are acting together rather than opposing each other. This seems self-evident, but you would be surprised how often you let your muscles work against each other rather than with each other. Pay attention to your body and see if you can recognize times when you can be more efficient!

The Barrel

Moving on from the idea of making a circle, here's another concept I greatly enjoy, and teach all my martial arts students. It's not something innately part of a martial arts discipline, but it helps the application. It also helps in everyday life. This concept is the "barrel." To see how this works, put your arms out in front of you, palms facing toward you, one hand behind the other, as if you're holding a giant barrel. You don't want the barrel to fall, so you have to keep up tension while you hold it.

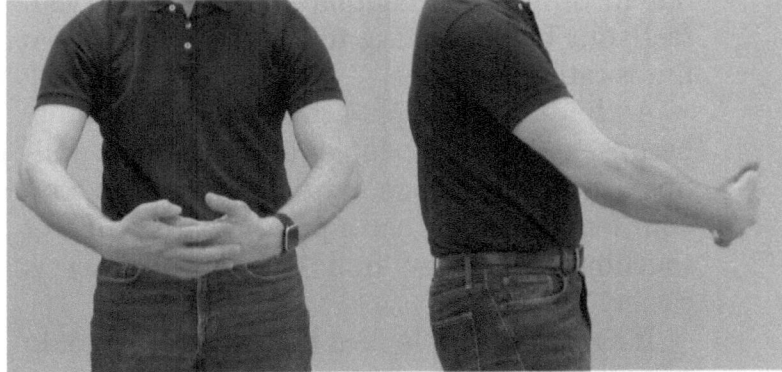

Figure 44: The "barrel." Hold your arms as if you are supporting a heavy pot or vase.

Ideally, you want to make the circle of your arms the same strength in every part. So, press out with your hands, your arms, your shoulders, and your back. You can test if your barrel is strong with somebody else's help. Have them randomly press on any part of the circle, and see if it collapses in. For a harder test, have them push against two opposing sides of your barrel, and see if it collapses. Often this will be at your elbows, or between your hands, or in the center of your back.

Why is the barrel important? This concept allows you to create a circle with your arms where force applied to them is deflected to the side. This means it's very hard to collapse. So what? Because you can use your arms when they are in "barrel form" to help you deflect incoming force. You can even keep the barrel going with only one hand. Go back to the example I showed you. Make a barrel out of your arms, then raise one hand higher and let the other one sink lower. You still have a barrel except your hands aren't actually touching. It's not as strong (because you're not completing a circle), but that doesn't always matter.

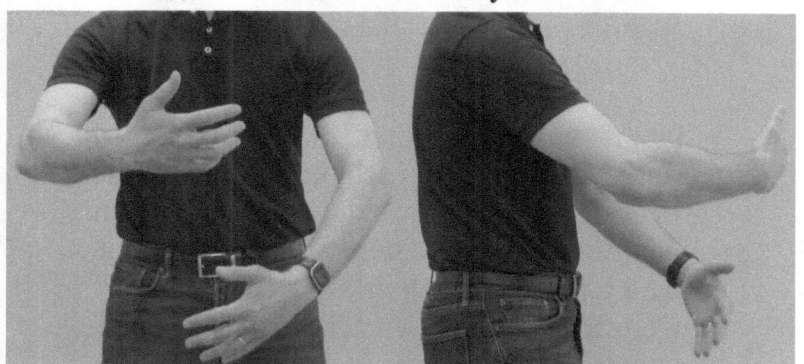

Figure 45: A separated barrel. There is less strength in this one, but more mobility.

Okay, here's a practical example. Find one of those big heavy metal doors with the press bar across them. Make a barrel with your dominant arm (or both together if you really want), then walk into the door (preferably on the bar section). Remember the theory! You never want your arm to collapse. In "barrel" your arm can take the load of your entire body walking into the door, pressing the release bar, and opening the door without collapsing. You can keep walking through the door with less reduction in your speed while doing so.

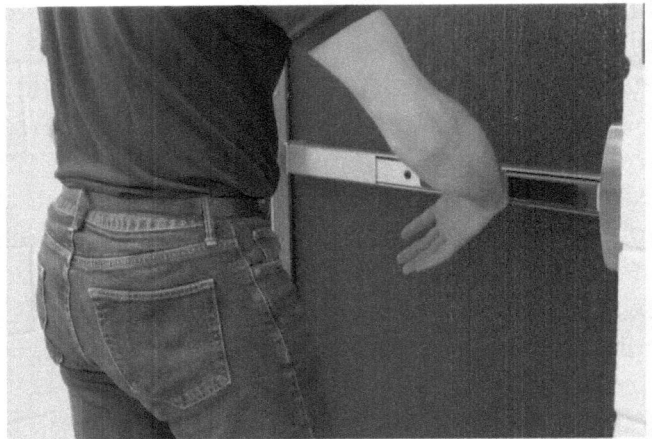

Figure 46: Using the barrel to open a door.

What if you're holding a heavy bag of groceries? Make a barrel with one arm to cradle the groceries against your side, or to hold them up by handle. This is the same idea as someone cradling a baby against their hip.

Don't want to touch a greasy banister in a public place? Try making a barrel with one arm and pressing the back of your wrist against the banister rather than holding it with your open hand.

You can get the same steadying feedback the banister is there for, but you don't have to touch it with a body part that is going to be touching (potentially) your mouth, nose, or eyes. Even though you aren't actively gripping the banister, you're still getting the kinesthetic feedback to tell you where you are in relation to it, and in relation to how the stairs slope downward. This isn't going to save you from tumbling down the stairs if you pitch forward, but it's likely to steady your balance enough so that you don't do so in the first place.

Here's an example of using the barrel with your legs. If you're on an unstable surface, like a moving vehicle or boat, try making a barrel with your lower half. It's the same idea, except your feet aren't going to be on top of each other, obviously. Instead, think about pressure through your knees. You want pressure down and around the outsides of your legs, so that your feet start to rest on the outside "ridge" edge.

You can feel this sort of stance is the same as making a barrel with your arms. You'll have to bend your knees when you do it, but then, you should never have your knees locked out anyway. You will resist motion sideways to your body. If that doesn't resist the motion in the correct direction, put one foot about two of your foot lengths in front of the other. Then press out with the front leg and back with the rear leg, sort of like what we did in the isometrics warm-up. This has the effect of creating a barrel-oriented front-to-rear of your

I described using the ridge edge in the section on "wobbling" and in the anatomy section. Yes, I'm finally getting to that explanation, but not quite all of it!

body rather than side-to-side. Depending on the direction of the motion you're dealing with, this stance should enable you to stay much more balanced.

There are a bunch of different applications for the barrel, which is why I like teaching it. Play around with it, with both your arms and your legs, and see if it helps you out too.

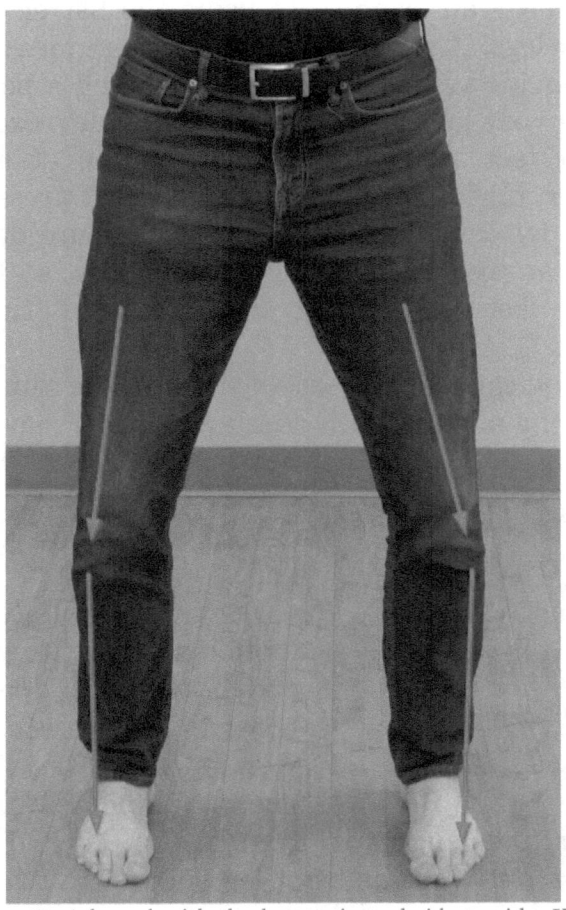

Figure 47: A barrel with the legs, oriented side to side. When attempting this you should feel pressure on the outside of your legs and feet.

Walking through doors

This is a corollary to the above section on the barrel, and it's a cool efficiency of movement I employ nearly every day. How do you walk smoothly through a door rather than pausing to open and close it? This is going to be a little complicated to explain, but it's also the end of the book. You're an expert now!

You're going to be using all four of your extremities when you do this. Let's start with going through a door that opens away from you rather than toward you. First, make a barrel with the arm that's going to open the door. Grip the door handle as you come close, but don't stop walking. Instead, keep your arm barreled and since you now walk with your center of mass moving forward in good posture, you can use your entire momentum to open the door as you walk through it.

> You can use a regular wood door in your house, so you don't have to exert yourself pushing a release bar.

You may need to walk around the door slightly as it opens. But that's not all! Keep holding on to the handle, and once you're through the doorway, you can push on the handle, or move your hand to grab the edge of the door, while still keeping the barrel in your arm. Then shut the door behind you as you move through it. It's all one motion. You don't have to stop, push open the door, walk through the doorway, turn around, and push the door closed.

154 William C. Tracy

Now let's try this with a door that swings toward you. This is slightly more complex, because you have to pass the door from one hand to the other. Instead, pull on the door, and use the momentum of pulling the door toward you (covered in "muscles moving against each other") to step past it as it swings open. Next you will need to pass the door from the hand that opened it to your other hand, which should be behind you as you move through the doorway. Keep walking forward, and let your rear hand pull the door closed as you do so. Again, pretty much all one motion: open the door, pass through it, and close it behind you. If you don't want to close the door, you can instead let it continue to open behind you.

You may need to slow down for this one on the approach to the door. Make sure you can grip the handle and pull it toward you, rather than opening the door directly into your face (not a desired outcome).

If you get good at this action, it makes moving through doorways very quick. Try it out with public bathroom stalls, because the doors are often spring-loaded, and close a lot more easily. But because you're in a confined space, you may need to use your newfound turning ability now you have excellent posture and are not slinging your center of mass around as you turn. There's plenty of space to turn between a stall door and a toilet, isn't there?

Walking sideways

We've come to the last section for this book. We've covered a *lot* of ground (mentally and physically). There's much more I want to tell you about, but it will have to wait for another book. We've only covered the lower half of the body, after all. There are plenty of other joints and muscles to investigate!

For now, I'm going to bring in an astonishing concept. Did you know your legs move sideways as well as forward and backward? This, *finally*, is what I wanted to talk about way back when I was explaining how your feet moved. But we needed all that explanation in the middle before I could explain it properly. So here it is.

What's the first step? Yes, that's right, good posture. If you're slumping for this one, it's not going to work as well. Stand up straight, then rather than taking a step forward, take a step to the side. Bend both knees a little bit and try to land just slightly on the outside ridge edges of your feet rather than flat. This is similar to rolling heel-toe, except you're going side-side. Lift up one foot just enough so it clears your other foot, move it across your standing leg, either in front or in back, and move your center of balance with it. If you stop at the midpoint of the step with your legs crossed, they will be crossed around your knee height, both knees will be bent, and both feet will be planted on the outside ridge. Continue moving your center to the side, bring your other foot around, and plant it flat on the floor. Congratulations, you've just stepped sideways.

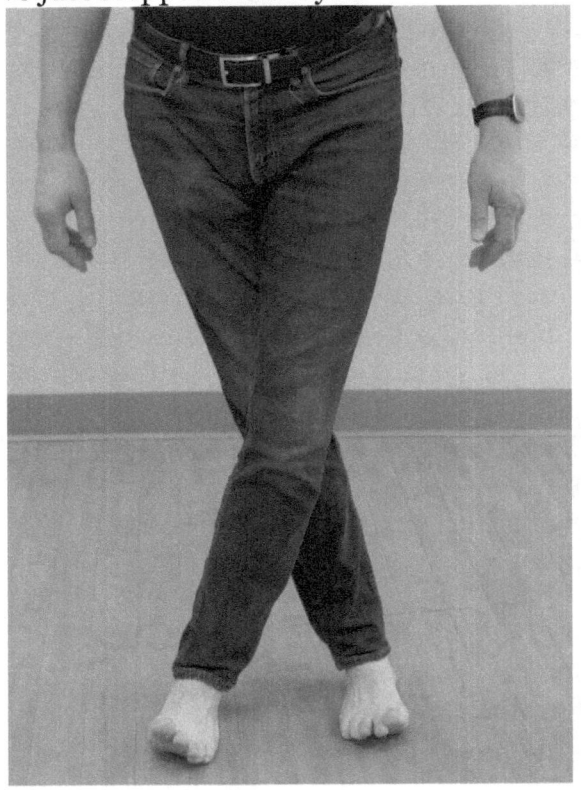

Figure 48: Stepping sideways on the ridge-edge of the feet.

Try this with your foot stepping across in *front* of your stationary leg and also *behind* your stationary leg, because you're going to use both ways. Attempt this sequence slowly to get used to stepping in a different direction than normal. Once you get some confidence in it, try stepping first in front of your stationary foot, and then behind your (new) foot when you take the next step. Once you get good at it, it's almost as fast to walk sideways as it is to walk forward, especially if you're taking advantage of good posture to keep your center of mass where it's supposed to be.

But you're not going to be walking sideways all the time. Where is something like this useful? For me, the counter in my kitchen is laid out in a line, from the fridge, to the sink, to the stove. There are shelves above with cooking products. So, when I'm using the kitchen, rather than turn sideways and slumping along the counter until I get where I want to be, I simply step sideways. Say I'm washing a bowl in the sink. Finish washing, dry it off, step sideways to the correct cabinet, open it up (using your barrel, right?), bowl in, door closed, step sideways back to where I need to be.

But don't just take my examples as the only thing you can do with these tips and tricks. Play around with. Do them so much they are encoded in your muscle memory. Then, when you do an unfamiliar action, one of these might come out, whether it's using a barrel, or walking sideways, or using one muscle against another for better effect.

In fact, that might be the main takeaway from this book. Even if you didn't do the exercises (but you did do them all, didn't you?), you should still have a better understanding of how your body works. Hopefully some of these ideas have sunk in, and one or two of them might come out and surprise you one of these days.

Wrap-up

Well, that was a lot! Congratulations on learning how to operate your body. Or, should I say, learning how to operate *part* of your body. The core concept of this book was simply how to walk. While that's most of what you use your legs for, it's certainly not all. And I haven't even touched on how to operate your arms, your hands, and your head!

If you have gone through the exercises, I hope you've learned a lot about the way your body works. Simply standing up straight is a big step to easing back, knee, and other joint pain. While I go on about moving efficiently, moving *correctly* is just as important. I see a lot of people in pain while they move around. I see a lot of others who don't necessarily have joint pain, but I can tell their body will degrade faster because they are not using it properly. You've taken a big step in coming this far.

> If you like the examples in this book, I've put together a series of videos along with the other teachers at my martial arts school. We take these concepts, and some others I haven't covered, in three-to-five-minute clips. If you've enjoyed this book, I think you'll enjoy them too. You can find them here: https://www.youtube.com/@howtooperateyourbody6460

I think it's safe to say there will be more where this came from. I can help you, but only if you take the time to learn what I've shown here. Just imagine learning how to operate your feet, legs, arms, hands, and head! If you do that, there is a whole other series of actions that you can do with your entire body, rather than just part of it.

Remember, practice makes perfect. That's a trite saying, but it became a cliché because it's true. I touched on muscle memory during this book, and it's actually a big part of how you live your daily life. You don't think about how every little muscle moves until you start learning a new skill. Then you suddenly become aware of whatever body part you're using to do that new skill.

I want you to get to a place where you're constantly questioning how your body moves, and never falling into a routine. Even if you've committed good posture to muscle memory, and you think you always stand up straight, take a second or two to check every once in a while. You may find your body has tricked you and decided to go back to some old habit. This can be frustrating and feels like you're taking a step backward rather than forward. The fact that you noticed it means you're learning! So don't despair. Because there

I also run an online workshop where I will personally teach you how to operate your body. Just go to my Patreon page at https://www.patreon.com/wctracy
Think of it like reading this book, but you can ask me questions while you're doing it, and I can tell you all the things I forgot or didn't have time to put in here.

isn't a convenient manual, it takes a lifetime to truly learn how to operate your body. Your success is measured by every single step you take, forward, back, or sideways. Your success is measured by *doing* it, rather than by ignoring your body, and hoping it stops bothering you. Keep at it.

I hope you liked this book. If you learned even one new thing, I'll count that as a success. I love teaching, because every so often I see that look on a student's face that tells me they've *got* it. If you have that same epiphany, please let me know. You can email me at wctracy@williamctracy.com. In addition, if you thought you gained something from this book, please leave a review at the bookseller where you purchased it. You'll be helping other people make the same decision you did and take the first step in learning How to Operate Your Body.

One more option! I teach all this in my martial arts class. If you live in North Carolina, and are interested in joining my school, I welcome anyone who is interested in changing their life for the better. You can find more information here: https://www.meetup.com/Raleigh-Wado-Ryu-Karate/

ACKNOWLEDGEMENTS

I'm a writer, an engineer, and a martial artist. Sometimes, I have to be told not to stare at people when they let me out of the house. I'm either staring because the person will make a great character in a book, or because I'm trying to understand how they're interacting with the world and using/misusing some piece of technology, or because some part of the way they walk has caught my attention. You'd be surprised how often it's the last one. Eventually, I decided to write a book about it.

Thanks first go to my co-teachers, Josiah and Courtney Brooks, for helping with concepting this book and developing the online videos for How to Operate Your Body (or as we fondly call it, HTOYB). As we've taught martial arts, we've found it matters less the system you start with, and more how the human body moves. We've all got the same basic body concept, and understanding how joints and muscles move means understanding the possibilities that we don't always take advantage of.

I want to thank all my fellow martial artists as well, both peers and students. I've learned many times more while teaching than practicing on my own. Also thank you Scott, Greg, and TJ for some early examples of how not to walk ;-)

Thanks as always to my beta readers, who tell me when I'm not making any sense, and lastly, but never least, to my copy editor (and wife) Heather for fixing all my writing mistakes.

ABOUT THE AUTHOR

William C. Tracy writes and publishes queer science fiction and fantasy through his indie press Space Wizard Science Fantasy (spacewizardsciencefantasy.com).

His largest work is the Dissolutionverse: a science fantasy series about planets connected by music-based magic instead of spaceflight. He also has an epic fantasy about a land where magic comes from seasonal fruit, and two sisters plot to take down a corrupt government. He is currently writing a space colony trilogy set on a planet entirely covered by a sentient fungus.

William is a North Carolina native with a master's in mechanical engineering, and has both designed and operated heavy construction machinery. He has trained in Wado-Ryu karate since 2003, and runs his own dojo in Raleigh, NC. In his spare time, he cosplays with his wife, and they enjoy putting their pets in cute little costumes and making them pose for the annual Christmas card.

Follow him on Bluesky @wctracy.bsky.social, Twitter @wctracy, or on Mastodon at wandering.shop/@wctracy for writing updates, cat and bee pictures, thoughts on martial arts, and new releases from his small press. Visit him online at www.spacewizardsciencefantasy.com or www.patreon.com/wctracy.

Please take a moment to review this book at your favorite retailer's website, Goodreads, or simply tell your friends!